10.95

MODERN MEDICAL MISTAKES

Edward C. Lambert, M.D.

Indiana University Press
Bloomington and London

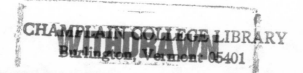

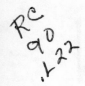

Manufactured in Canada

Library of Congress Cataloging in Publication Data

Lambert, Edward C.
  Modern medical mistakes.

  Bibliography: p.

  1. Iatrogenic diseases — History. 2. Therapeutics — Complications and sequelæ — History. 3. Drugs — Side effects — History. I. Title. [DNLM: 1. Malpractice. 2. Medication errors. W44 L222m]
RC90.L35   615'.5   77-15214
ISBN 0-253-15425-1

"To judge rightly on the present we must oppose it to the past; for all judgment is comparative, and of the future nothing can be known. . . . The present state of things is the consequence of the former, and it is natural to inquire what were the sources of the good that we enjoy, or the evil that we suffer. If we act only for ourselves, to neglect the study of history is not prudent; if we are entrusted with the care of others it is not just."

Rasselas, Chapter 30
Samuel Johnson

Foreword

This book, the fascinating story of major errors in medical treatment of the twentieth century and of how they were detected, is for everyone, not just for doctors. It was written in lucid and non-technical prose by Dr. Edward C. Lambert, one of the most beloved and respected leaders of American Medicine.

Speaking to doctors and patients alike, Dr. Lambert says that if this book "only teaches the reader awareness of the hazard of unnecessary treatment and the need for critical evaluation of new remedies, it will have served a useful purpose." He cites numerous examples of non-essential or ineffective remdies that led to death or deformity and deplores "the foolish but persistent belief that health and wellbeing can be purchased and maintained by medication or surgery." Although Dr. Lambert agrees with Benjamin Franklin's observation that "nothing is more fatal to health than an overcare of it," and with Sir William Osler's dictum that "one of the first duties of the physician is to educate the masses not to take medicine," he adds that, in fairness, "many physicians need to be educated not to prescribe unnecessarily."

Regarding the evaluation of new remedies, Dr. Lambert states that well-designed controlled clinical trials are necessary in order to decide whether a treatment is truly effective. He welcomes the healthy humility at last being developed by physicians and observes that "the doctrine of professorial infallibility, the arrogant, authoritarian, autocratic attitude so common among successful academic physicians and surgeons, is disappearing in the western world and is being replaced by a willingness to submit all treatments to critical tests." Dr. Lambert considers not only the medical but also the ethical aspects of a properly done trial of treatment, insisting that "the safety and well-being of the patient must always be the chief consideration."

Dr. Lambert concludes that the 'doctor's dilemma' is not the choice of whom to save, as it was in Shaw's play. Rather it is the dilemma that every doctor faces daily, with varying success, of how to treat and help without harming. "The Hippocratic admonition, 'first do no harm'," he feels "cannot strictly apply. Risks must be taken if benefits are to be maximal. Few risks are justified when the illness is minor and self-limited. Major risks may be justified when the illness is major, death likely, and no simple effective treatment is available."

This unique book is not only a tale of major medical errors and their detection; it is also a philosophy of modern Medicine for doctors and patients alike.

People in all walks of life were proud to claim Dr. Edward C. Lambert as a friend. This book was written during 1973 when he was on sabbatical in London, England. He was the Director of the Division of Cardiology of the Children's Hospital of Buffalo, New York, until his untimely death in March of 1974 at fifty-eight years of age. He was the author of more than sixty scientific publications. This book is Dr. Lambert's last work — his only one for the general reader. It may well be his greatest.

RICHARD VAN PRAAGH, M.D.
Children's Hospital Medical Center
Harvard Medical School
Boston, Massachusetts

Preface

In medical school, as an intern and a resident, and as a pediatrician, I observed and participated in new methods of treatment which have been gratifying and exciting — the use of sulfa drugs and antibiotics, the cure of rickets and scurvy in infants, the prevention of polio, the advances in cardiac surgery. But I was also a party to several forms of treatment which resulted in much unnecessary misery. Several years ago it occurred to me that the story of modern mistakes of treatment was largely untold. Bits and pieces of it are scattered about. But the books on medical history, except for those relating to the specialties, leave this story out.

I believed, and many of my colleagues agreed, that it was a story worth telling, with many lessons. I have told it simply and from the point of view of a practicing doctor.

What began as a narrative account developed into a critical study of the methods of evaluation of forms of therapy and the manner in which they are accepted and discarded. It will be apparent that more recent events are stressed, and more space is given to matters involving the English and Americans. This reflects in part my lack of knowledge about medical practice in other parts of the world; in part, the audience for whom this work is intended — men and women, professional and non-professional, of the English-speaking world, who are curious about the healing arts.

Friends have advised me that this account may upset and antagonize some of my colleagues. This is in no way my intent. The accomplishments of modern medicine have been so magnificent that we as a profession should be able to admit mistakes gracefully. The public needs to understand the nature of and the need for trials of treatments and the folly and hazards of seeking and using unnecessary medication.

10

Introduction

"There are some patients whom we cannot help: there are none whom we cannot harm." Bloomfield

The twentieth century is the Age of Therapy. Effective treatment and prevention of disease in the individual began this century, and progress has been greater, more significant, and more decisive than in all previous time. The foundations had been laid by the great bacteriologists, biochemists, pathologists and physiologists of the last half of the 1800s.

In previous centuries, on the whole, more patients were harmed than were cured by the remedies used by the doctors. Lawrence Henderson, the famous biochemist and medical historian at Harvard, stated that not until about 1911 did the random patient consulting the random physician begin to have a better than even chance of being helped.

From the small number of effective drugs available at the turn of the century, the present therapeutic armamentarium has expanded to several thousand. Antibiotics, vaccines, antihypertensive agents, psychotropic drugs, x-ray, electrolyte solutions, endocrines and vitamins, together with public health measures, have contributed greatly to the well-being of Man and have increased his life-expectancy past middle age. Pestilence in the forms of plague, malaria, smallpox, yellow fever, polio, tuberculosis and other infections has been controlled. Advances in surgery and post-operative care have dramatically contributed to the quality and the length of life of those to whom such are available economically and geographically.

None the less, these advances have been accompanied by a host of iatrogenic (physician-produced) diseases, usually as side effects. They have been referred to as the "diseases of medical progress."

11

In addition, errors of concept based on wrong ideas have led to both useless and often harmful methods of treatment. It seems possible that a review of these recent errors may help us to better judge the present.

This is the account of selected treatments in which, on a large scale, the harm done outweighed the benefits. In each instance, strong circumstantial evidence of either lack of effectiveness or tragic results led to the treatment's being modified, replaced, or abandoned. The list is by no means exhaustive, but most of the outstanding examples which involved many doctors and more patients are included. It is possible that certain of the errors considered here may not be considered such in the future; there is the danger of their being too close in time for needed perspective. Some treatments, such as bleeding, which extended into the century, are left out.

The story of quackery has been told many times and does not belong here. The madness or eccentricity of individual doctors productive of such treatments as Krebiozen or Abram's black box had little impact on other physicians, and also do not seem appropriate in this account. Toxic or unpleasant side effects of useful drugs should not be accounted errors. Finally, while the many individual abuses of well-founded forms of treatment — medical and surgical — probably account for more needless suffering, they appear to be another problem altogether. With the peculiar exceptions of surgery and medical treatment performed in relation to the theories of focal infection and of autointoxication, such abuses are not considered.

The rest is the story of disasters and scandals, follies, suffering and death, epidemics and endemic diseases, and unnecessary surgery involving tens of thousands of people — all as a result of treatments undertaken by honourable, often distinguished, physicians with the best of intentions. Deliberately, it is a narrow, one-sided analysis of aspects of some of the problems of therapy; for during the same period millions have been helped, cured, or prevented from developing disease.

Though most doctors who care for patients are aware of many of the errors analyzed here and have committed some of them, few know them all, or their details. Works on the history of medicine are surprisingly lacking in accounts of our mistakes in this century as compared with previous ones. This is the dark side of the ledger of our time, which is largely omitted from the histories.

We have learned by our mistakes in the past and will continue to learn in the future. The lessons learned and the changes made are the heartening side of the story. These changes have already reduced the chances of similar errors occurring again on such a scale. However, if this review only teaches the reader awareness of the hazard of unnecessary treatment and the need for critical evaluation of new remedies, it will have served a useful purpose.

The errors are classified as those of concept, those due to laboratory mistakes and accidents, drug side effects, and drug overdose. These divisions are not absolute and are largely for convenience. Several items could have equally well been put into another category. In addition, a chapter has been added which includes four examples of possible errors in whch a mistake was not proven.

At the outset, it is useful to consider the specific application in this presentation of some of the terms fundamental in any consideration of treatment. The terms which are used repeatedly are: control, disease, double blind, drug, epidemic, idiosyncracy, placebo and randomization.

Control — a standard for comparison. The controlled trial is the basis for the evaluation of the effects of a treatment, beneficial or harmful, about which there exists doubt. It is performed in order to obtain definitive, objective evidence. The care of the patients should be the same in all respects, except for the one factor being studied. Similarly, the group used as controls — animal or human, as the case may be — must match as closely as possible with respect to such important factors as age, sex, severity of disease, duration of illness, etc. Both groups should be cared for at the same time. Finally, and of equal importance, the number of subjects involved must be sufficient to preclude the possibility of the results occurring by chance.

Disease ("lack of ease") — any illness or malady, or a characteristic group of symptoms or physical findings on examination.

Double-blind — a technique used in controlled trials by which the emotional attitudes and prejudices — skepticism as well as enthusiasms — of both the patients and the physicians evaluating them are avoided until the test is over. Neither the patients nor the doctors observing the results know the nature of the treatment; both are "blind". In addition, the doctors should have no knowledge or choice in the allocation of patients to the control or to the treated groups.

Drug — any chemical substance whatsoever (gas, solid or liquid, other than food) used in any way for medical purposes — prevention, treatment, or diagnosis. In this context, vaccines, vitamins, and oxygen are drugs.

Epidemic ("upon the people") — once used to refer only to contagious illnesses involving many people. Now it refers to any increase in the frequency of a disease or condition in a population in excess of normal expectation. Epidemiology involves the study of disease in populations, by the application of statistics with determination of probabilities. Factors such as age, sex, geographic distribution, season, timing, local customs, and medical histories are considered, together with the possibilities of control of the disease or condition.

Idiosyncracy — in an individual, a reaction to a drug completely different from that shown by the vast majority of the same species.

Placebo (" I will please") — originally used to refer to any inactive substance used for psychological effect only. Now used broadly to apply to any sham or dummy medication or procedure considered to have only psychological effect, and substituted in the control group for the medication or procedure tested, to which it must be identical in appearance. It is a powerful tool which can bring about ill effects as well as cures. Controlled studies may compare two methods of treatment, or one method may be compared with a placebo.

Randomization — the assignment of subjects to treatment and control groups on a chance basis, so that each has an equal probability of being chosen for any one of the groups being compared. A basic feature of trials, employed to eliminate bias and prejudice in selection on the part of the investigators, and to insure as far as possible that the patients in each group are similar in all respects relevant to the study.

CHAPTER ONE

Errors of Concept

"A beautiful theory killed by nasty, ugly little facts."

T. H. Huxley

Theories and concepts of anatomy, physiology, biochemistry, and mechanisms of disease have more strongly influenced medical treatment in this century than in previous ones. The nineteenth century brought an explosion of research in the fields of physics, biochemistry and physiology, and the development of the new sciences of bacteriology and immunology. These became the bases for many new approaches to disease. Because of anesthesia, surgery became painless; because of control of infections, it became safe, resulting in the disappearance of previous reluctance to resort to it. Advances in chemistry permitted the synthesis of a myriad of drugs. The new ideas, together with availability of many new treatments, led to impressive achievements in the new conquest of disease — and to follies and abuses.

Three concepts — autointoxication, vaccine therapy, and focal infection — affected the thinking and practice of most doctors and led to a variety of unnecessary or harmful treatments during the first half of the century. The other six concepts presented here resulted in single specific forms of treatment for specific common conditions. All were abandoned because new evidence failed to support the concepts, and because the results were more harmful than beneficial.

Autointoxication

Man has been obsessed with his bowels since earliest days. The Ebers Papyrus, written in the sixteenth century B.C., advises that

15

if a few seeds of the ricinus plant (from which castor oil is obtained) are "chewed with beer by a person who is constipated it will expel the stool from the body of that person." (Castor oil may have been the first effective drug known to man.) The Papyrus also mentions giving enemas up to three pints. Later, Herodotus tells us that the Egyptians tried to be clean internally by evacuating the intestinal tract for three consecutive days every month. The word cathartic derives from the Greek "to cleanse," indicating the idea of cleaning the body internally by ridding it of its waste products. "Purge," from the Latin, has the same meaning.

Down through the ages, feces have been considered dirty, foul, unhealthy, impure. The term catharsis was applied by analogy to the mind, to indicate purification of the passions. The English term "physic" is used both for cathartics and for medicines in general, hence the term "physician."

Well into the nineteenth century purging, along with medicines to induce vomiting and bleeding, was one of the most common forms of treatment for many complaints, and the source of most medical satire. In the middle ages, the use of voluminous medicated enemas, termed clysters, was customary. In the *Imaginary Invalid,* Molière addresses "the vain and foolish doctors" of his time. The play opens with Argan, the hypochondriac, reading his doctor's bill. "Item, on the twenty-fourth, a small injection preparatory, insinuative, and emollient, to lubricate, loosen, and stimulate the gentleman's bowels . . . to flush, irrigate, and thoroughly clean out the gentleman's lower intestine: thirty sous." On the stage, the action is enhanced by the flourish of giant clyster syringes. (These syringes are still present in some of Daumier's bitter political cartoons in the nineteenth century.) In 1727 Jonathan Swift imparted some of his scorn of the human animal in the description of the habits of his fellow countrymen given by Gulliver to the Houyhnhnms: "They take in at the orifice above a medicine equally annoying and disgustful to the bowels, which relaxing the belly drives down all before it; and this they call a purge."

Near the end of the nineteenth century, theories and ideas relating to disorders of the intestinal tract were upgraded, made more complex, respectable and sophisticated, by borrowings from the scientific contributions of the great physiologists, bacteriologists, biochemists and pathologists of the time. Two related concepts were proposed — visceroptosis and autointoxication. They were made to account for a variety of complaints (loss of appetite, nausea, asthenia, depression, "pains in the midship section," backache, insomnia, chronic invalidism) which, taken together, were thought to indicate one disease. The patient was usually described as thin and flabby, with poor posture and a protuberant abdomen, the skin muddy, the pupils dilated, the respirations rapid and frequently irregular.

The concept of visceroptosis — a prolapse or falling of the intestines and the other abominal organs — was proposed by a French physician, Glénard, who wrote some thirty papers about the problem. The concept aroused much interest and controversy. By 1912, according to one reviewer, more than a thousand medical articles on the subject had appeared, many enthusiastic, some skeptical. The condition came to be called Glénard's disease. In its original simple form, the theory postulated that the long intestines cramped in the abdominal cavity became kinked if the contents of a loop of intestines were too large or too little. Stasis (a favourite term) resulted. The loss of gas from the partially obstructed bowel was thought to remove support from the stomach, liver, spleen, kidneys, and even the uterus, causing them to drop because of man's erect posture. (The corsets worn by women were believed to add to the problem.) In its original form, Glénard's concept was a mechanical one.

Near the turn of the century the theory of autointoxication — self poisoning — was superimposed on the ideas of visceroptosis. This theory postulated that, as a result of stasis, putrefaction of the intestinal contents occurred; toxins were formed and absorbed, leading to chronic poisoning of the body. Various breakdown products of enzymatic action of the bacteria in the colon were identified as toxins. In 1903 both concepts were taken up and elaborated on by one of the most famous, skilful, original, and indefatigable surgeons of the time, Sir William Arbuthnot Lane, Senior Surgeon at both Guys Hospital and at the Hospital for Sick Children, Great Ormond Street, London. Lane's versatility was such that he devised useful techniques for the treatment of fractures, harelip and cleft palate, acute intestinal obstruction, and infections of the mastoid.

Surgeons came from Europe and North and South America to watch him operate at Guys. Conan Doyle was later to admit that Lane, because of his powers of observation and qualities of personality, was one of the models for the character of Sherlock Holmes. In 1911, at the World Congress of Surgery in New York, Sir Arbuthnot was given a standing ovation. In a series of seventy-five papers published over a twenty-five year period, he persuasively argued his theories of chronic intestinal stasis and its toxic effects. In the United States and France, Glénard's disease became Lane's disease. His beliefs were supported by the theories of the famous Russian zoologist and Nobel prizewinner, Ilya Mechnikov, who believed that the large intestine (the colon) was a vestigial organ like the appendix, of no value, and a source of trouble to Man. At first Lane performed a short-circuiting operation to connect the lower end of the small intestine and the far end of the large (ileosigmoidostomy), thus by-passing most of the colon. Later, with the encouragement of Mechnikov, he performed a colectomy — removal of the entire colon. In his enthusiasm and eagerness, Lane, and many others, were led to believe that this surgery was also of value in the treatment of duodenal ulcer, bladder disease, rheumatoid arthritis, tuberculosis, schizophrenia, high blood pressure, arteriosclerosis, and in the prevention of cancer of the intestinal tract. He performed with great skill, resulting in low mortality, more than a thousand colectomies, often observed by enthusiastic audiences of fellow surgeons. In England his theories were for the most part received with skepticism and hostility, but were accepted by many in the United States and on the continent. Colectomy was a much performed operation.

Though Bernard Shaw denied it, many thought that Cutler Walpole, the prosperous, aggressive surgeon in *Doctors Dilemma,* was Lane. Here is Walpole: "Ninety-five per cent of the human race suffer from chronic blood-poisoning and die of it. It's as simple as A.B.C. Your nuciform sac is full of decaying matter — undigested food and waste products — rank ptomaines. Now you take my advice, Ridgeon. Let me cut it out for you. You'll be another man afterwards."

A variation was the diagnosis of colitis, or, sometimes, mucous colitis. This diagnosis assumed that an inflamed or irritated colon explained the abdominal pains, backache, malaise, chronic invalidism, and the mucous often present in the stool. The proponents of visceroptosis and of autointoxication argued that their concepts explained the basis for colitis and that it was but one aspect of the problem. Colitis became an extremely fashionable diagnosis, particularly among the wealthy women of Paris just before the First World War. In a best-selling novel of the twenties and thirties, *The Story of San Michele,* the physician Axel Munthe gives a vivid picture of the popularity of the diagnosis and its remarkable value in masking the ignorance of the doctor.

The Scottish physician in Aldous Huxley's novel, *Eyeless in Gaza,* expresses a common professional attitude of the twenties and early thirties, and the preoccupation with indigestion and autointoxication: "How can you expect to think in anything but a negative way, when you've got chronic intestinal poisoning? Had it from birth, I guess. Inherited it. And at the same time stooping as you do. Pressing down on the vertabrae like a ton of bricks. One can almost hear the poor things grinding together. And when the spine's in that state, what happens to the rest of the machine? It's frightful to think of. . . . Speaking as a doctor, I'd suggest a course of colonic irrigation to start with. . . . Only a proper diet. No butcher's meat; it's poison, so far as you're concerned. And milk; it'll only blow you up with wind."

Another school developed a cross-over between the theory of autointoxication and that of focal infection, another concept discussed in this chapter. In place of chemical toxins entering the blood stream from the intestines, its proponents substituted bacteria and made the colon and appendix other foci. Both schools subscribed to the idea of chronic appendicitis — stasis in the appendix, producing continual release of toxins or of bacteria. This led to the unnecessary removal of many thousands of normal appendices.

An offshoot of the visceroptosis concept was the belief in the existence of undue mobility of the first portion of the colon, causing it to wander with change in position, producing abdominal pains and recurrent vomiting. This was corrected by anchoring it in its proper place (ceco-colon fixation).

As a result of these theories and concepts, seven types of operations were performed on many thousands of people, few of whom were benefited more than temporarily. Many were made worse;

some died. These operations included the following, most of which are useful today when there are appropriate indications for them:

Colectomy and hemi-colectomy

Ceco-colon fixation

Gastropexy (This consisted of shortening a stomach previously lengthened by being pulled down. It was done to permit the stomach to empty by gravity.)

Fixation of the uterus

Fixation of the kidney

Appendectomy for chronic appendicitis

In addition to these surgical procedures, there existed medical treatments for the most part derived from the previous centuries. Lane himself, anxious to prevent chronic intestinal stasis and the use of harsh cathartics, advised an abdominal belt and liberal amounts of mineral oil. For years he dosed himself with this laxative oil. Others, patients and doctors, kept themselves regular — one or two bowel movements a day — by use of roughage in the diet, or by regular daily laxatives of all sorts. "Regularity" became a moral virtue for those who desired internal cleanliness. Enemas were expanded to colonic irrigations — up to thirty pints of fluid given over a two-hour period. At the expensive spas in England and on the continent, these irrigations were euphemistically spoken of as "intestinal lavage." In the United States, they were administered at "colon laundries." Children were often given a "high colonic" by their parents, as a general treatment for many complaints.

Unhappily, these medical treatments tended to perpetuate the very condition they were devised to treat. In addition to becoming irritated, the rectum and colon, emptied of their contents, naturally required more than the usual time to fill, before re-emptying in a normal fashion from normal stimuli. The patient, not aware of this, believed he was again becoming constipated, and without waiting, once more resorted to laxatives or enemas. A condition now called cathartic colon often resulted.

These abuses by doctors and patients alike appear to have reached their peak by the eve of the First World War. By then, many physicians — mainly internists and radiologists — appalled by these excesses, were gathering evidence which gradually led to the abandonment of the concepts of both visceroptosis and autointoxication, and to the realization that the constipation, the complaints, and the clinical findings were usually secondary to the emotional and psychic disturbances of the patient, and not due to mechanical problems of the abdominal contents nor to the absorption of toxins or bacteria. Nervous indigestion, appropriately, became the diagnosis. Briefly, the evidence was:

1. The discovery, largely by x-ray, of a wide variation in mobility and length of the intestinal tract in young, normal, healthy men and women. Obstructive kinks were not demonstrable in symptomatic patients.
2. The failure, in spite of repeated tests and analyses, to demonstrate chemical toxins in the blood which could account for the symptoms.*
3. The production of most of the symptoms — pains, malaise, headache, etc. — by mechanical distension of the rectum with cotton, suppositories, or barium.
4. The documentation of extreme variation in bowel habits among active individuals in good health and free of symptoms. Careful observation revealed that many persons normally have bowel movements only once or twice a week. An occasional healthy individual may go several weeks without one. Palmer stated: "Constipation should be defined as any condition that causes the patient to complain that his bowels are not moving enough or often enough. . . . One man's constipation is another man's diarrhea."
5. The repeated finding by careful observers that patients were not benefited more than temporarily by cathartics, colonic irrigations, and the wide variety of abdominal surgical procedures. Many were made worse. No controlled clinical trials were performed.

In spite of the fact that all this evidence was available and widely published by the mid-twenties, the abuses were slow to disappear. In 1935 Sir Arthur Hurst, an eminent English gastroenterologist, who had opposed most of Lane's views for twenty-five years,

---

*There are exceptions. Autointoxication with accumulation of toxins may occur rarely as a result of severe liver disease or advanced kidney failure.

21

spoke at Harvard "On the Unhappy Colon." In this lecture he felt impelled to comment with bitter humour, "The vast army of hypochondriacs, who are never happy unless their stools conform to an ideal which they have invented for themselves, can only be cured by making themselves realize that feces have no standard size, shape, consistency, or colour; they are then ready to follow the example of the dog rather than the cat — and never look behind them."

While the theories of visceroptosis and autointoxication were condemned in the textbooks and medical schools in the 1930s, the medical and surgical practices lingered on into the 1950s. Surgery for chronic appendicities and mobile colons was slow to disappear. Hospitals instituted committees to periodically review the number of normal appendices removed, in order to minimize unnecessary operations. Health spas turned to other less uncomfortable forms of treatment. The colon laundries closed their doors. While laxatives and cathartics of all types still enjoy an enormous sale in Europe and America, a generation has grown up which is not bowel-conscious. Man has learned that the billions of bacteria which thrive on his skin and in his intestinal tract are for the most part not harmful, and may even be beneficial. Germ-free animals can be raised in artificial environments, but they lead a precarious existence and are highly susceptible to infections.

Vaccine Therapy

The successes in the prevention of human infectious diseases by the use of vaccines (killed or weakened viruses or bacteria) by Jenner and Pasteur led to the attempt to treat chronic or recurrent infections by a similar approach. This second error to be discussed here was almost entirely the concept of one person, an exceptionally talented and able Irishman, one of the outstanding bacteriologists of his time, Sir Almoth Wright. Wright devised the first effective method of inoculation to prevent typhoid fever, which saved thousands, originated many important bacteriologic tests and techniques, and established the profession of bacteriology in England.

In 1900 he hypothesized that therapeutic vaccination of the

already infected patient ought to work in spite of current arguments to the contrary. During the next two years he treated six patients with recurrent boils caused by staphlylococci, using heat-killed cultures of these bacteria secured from the infections of each patient. Like Sir Arbuthnot Lane, Wright was strongly influenced by Ilya Mechnikov, the founder of the important concept of cellular immunity. Twenty years before Mechnikov had described how invading bacteria were ingested and destroyed by the white cells in the blood, called phagocytes, and had postulated that this action was one of the important mechanisms in the body's defense against infection. Wright found that the capacity of the phagocytes to ingest bacteria was enhanced by the injection into the body of a specific vaccine prepared from the same bacteria which produced the infection. His measurement of this capacity he termed the phagocytic index. A high index indicated, he believed, an effective response.

All of the six patients improved over a period of several months, and their phagocytic indices rose. However, there was no good correlation between the clinical status of the patients and the ability of the phagocytes to take up the staphylococci. Also, the phagocytic indices were poorly reproducible, fluctuating wildly from time to time. Wright described the results of these experiments in *The Lancet* in 1902, and in this paper speculated optimistically on extensions of this approach to the therapy of tuberculosis, streptococcal infections, and gonorrhea. This publication began the era of vaccine therapy, which extended through the first half of the century and became a fashionable method of treating almost any disease. It was used widely by the believers in focal infection.

Sir Almoth was a tireless, forceful and eloquent advocate of his theory. Clinical departments of bacteriology were established in many hospitals in England, Europe, and the United States, in order to determine phagocytic (later refined to opsonic) indices and to prepare vaccines grown from the patients' own bacteria. Some good results were claimed in appendicitis, colitis, meningitis, as well as infections of the kidney, middle ear, uterus, and even recurrent colds. Wright stressed the special value of vaccine therapy in local forms of tuberculosis involving the skin, lymph nodes, kidney, bone, and peritoneum, using an extract of tubercle bacilli. He believed that it could be effective in pulmonary tuberculosis after the patient had been in bed sufficiently long for the temperature to return to normal. It was this application to tuberculosis which formed the basis for *Doctor's Dilemma*. Shaw used Sir Almoth Wright, his friend, as the prototype for Sir Colenso Ridgeon, the hero of the play. The dilemma relates to the choice, because of a limited supply of vaccine, of treating the good but elderly general practitioner, or the young, amoral, talented artist — both of them dying of tuberculosis. The decision had to be made as to "which life was the best worth saving." The phrase, "stimulate the phagocytes!" rings through the play. Rather than being flattered by Shaw's complimentary portrayal of him, Wright considered *The Doctor's Dilemma* a travesty of serious research and stalked out during its performance.

While Shaw ridiculed the ideas of autointoxication and the resulting wholesale removal of organs and other parts of the body thought to be useless or to harbour toxins, he was enthusiastic about vaccine therapy, which now appears equally ineffective though far less traumatic. Foster, in his excellent *History of Medical Bacteriology and Immunology,* points out that,

> For example, a rabbit could be immunized with a highly virulent streptococcus and it could be shown, experimentally, that not only would this particular rabbit withstand a dose of living streptococci, which would infallibly kill an unimmunized animal, but that the serum of the immune animal would passively protect a normal rabbit against challenge with the streptococcus. In the experimental situation, antibacterial serum therapy worked; the problems lay in transferring the principle to natural disease in man. These problems proved largely insoluble, but a great deal was learned in their investigation. However, with regard to vaccine therapy, the situation was quite different; no infected animal was ever convincingly cured of any bacterial disease by the administration of a vaccine. The evidence that vaccine therapy was a useful therapeutic procedure was derived from clinical work in man and would have been none the worse for that had it been evidence sufficient to convince a reasonable, critical and impartial observer. The trouble was that it was not.

Many individual examples were cited by Wright and others, of the benefits and apparent cures of specific cases. Clinical impressions of the value of vaccine therapy were often adduced; but no evidence lending itself to statistical analysis became available, and for many years there were no controlled clinical trials.

Sir Almoth in 1906 clearly expressed his opposition to planned controlled clinical trials carried on concurrently and subjected to statistical analysis such as that suggested by English statisticians:

> Now a series of untreated cases such as would serve th purpose of controls cannot in practical life be obtained. For such a series of untreated controls there would have to be substituted, as the only possible alternative, a series of cases treated by another method and by another practitioner. Now if this were done the scientific issue would be immediately confused, not only by doubts as to the comparability of the two series of cases, but also by the question as to whether the therapeutic method which was applied in the control series was hurtful, innocent, or beneficial; and above all it would be confused by a question of personal competition.
>
> If you will consider what confusion would in this way be introduced into the issue which we are here concerned to resolve, you will, I think, understand the motives which influence me when I say I do not propose, either here or elsewhere, to supplement by any attempted statistical proof that presumptive proof of the efficacy of vaccine-therapy which I claim to have already furnished by the citation of numerous refractory and desperate cases successfully treated by the inoculation of bacterial vaccines.

These words, delivered in an address at Johns Hopkins University, expressed not only Wright's feelings and attitude, but also those of most doctors toward almost any controlled trials employing patients, down through the first half of the present century. Later, Austin Bradford Hill and others were gradually able to convince many doctors that when there was doubt and ignorance about a new method of treatment, it was unethical *not* to test it appropriately by controlled studies. It was this disparaging attitude of Wright and others more than anything else, which perpetuated the mistakes of treatment through most of the present century. The tools were at hand, but they were not used at the time.

Even Frank Billings, professor of medicine and dean of Rush Medical School, the enthusiastic protagonist of focal infection, the concept discussed in the next section, had extreme difficulty with the determination of opsonic indices and failed to find vaccine therapy effective in a large series of cases. In the 1920s, clinicians and other bacteriologists became increasingly skeptical of the value of Wright's vaccines. Sir William Osler, the most influential clinician of the period, warned against "the wiles of that Celtic siren, Sir Almoth." In the 1930s, a carefully controlled study was carried out on a large number of patients with arthritis. They were divided into two equal groups at random. One group received weekly injections of carefully prepared vaccine; the other was given injections of saline. Just over two-thirds of the patients in each group were much improved. With the possible exception of recurrent boils from staphylococcal infections, in which the vaccines may act in a preventive rather than a therapeutic fashion, there is nothing now to indicate their value. Nevertheless, in spite of the condemnation by professors and textbook writers, these vaccines were not given up by physicians because of their lack of value; rather, they were merely, for the most part, replaced by the truly effective sulfonamides and antibiotics. Even in 1965 therapeutic vaccines for staphylococcal infections were produced by reputable firms and occasionally prescribed.

What harm was done? Little, other than the considerable expense to the patients and the discomfort from the injections. That "little," however, includes the occasional serious reaction or transmission of serum hepatitis and the rare death which may result from the use of any vaccine.

The substantial profits from the use and sales of the therapeutic vaccines made by Wright served a highly important function. They permitted the employment in 1921 of Alexander Fleming as Assistant Director of the Department of Therapeutic Inoculation at St. Mary's Hospital, London. It was there in 1929 that Fleming discovered the bactericidal effect of the penicillium mould producing penicillin. On the death of Sir Almoth in 1947, the Institute was renamed the Wright-Fleming Institute.

Focal Infection

The theory that localized pockets of bacterial infection around the teeth, tonsils, or other parts of the body produce or affect a wide variety of generalized diseases pervaded most of this century and led to more unnecessary surgery than did any other concept. It also engendered many foolish, unpleasant, and sometimes harmful medical practices. Almost all physicians between 1910 and 1950 were influenced by the theory, and even now the profession has not entirely escaped its effects, in spite of the fact that modern medical textbooks mention it only to condemn it.

Historically, the idea that infected teeth lead to other illness, especially rheumatism, was considered possible by the ancients, including Hippocrates. In more recent times, the flamboyant, erratic and influential American physician, Benjamin Rush, published in 1808 his observations suggesting that several chronic generalized diseases could be cured by removing infected teeth. He claimed to have cured a woman with arthritis of the hip by extracting her teeth. His ideas had little effect until shortly after the beginning of the present century, when the concept was revived and amplified with more enthusiasm and determination than proof.

Between 1910 and 1915 the American, Frank Billings, together with an outstanding English pathologist, William Hunter, proposed the plausible medical theory of focal infection. Billings was supported by an industrious bacteriologist, Edward Rosenow. The establishment in the second half of the nineteenth century of the germ theory of disease by Louis Pasteur and Robert Kach, followed by the identification of the specific organisms responsible for tuberculosis, cholera, plague, diphtheria, typhoid fever, and other infectious diseases, led to the search for bacteria which could account for many chronic diseases and ailments of unknown cause. It was commonly thought that the causes for most diseases were about to be discovered. The normal abundance of bacteria of many types in the mouth, nose, throat, intestinal tract, and genital tract offered exciting possibilities. The examples of gonorrhea, tuberculosis, and subacute bacterial endocarditis gave support to the idea that many chronic diseases could be due to localized low-grade bacterial infection. Gonorrheal arthritis is secondary to infection located in the genital tract. In tuberculosis of the bones, the primary site is most often the lung. The best example is that of subacute bacterial endocarditis in which a strain of streptococcus of low virulence, often primarily located in or around an infected tooth or tonsil, invades the blood stream and locates on a damaged heart valve, producing a prolonged and, if untreated, usually fatal illness characterized by recurrent fever. Further, it could be shown that extraction of tonsils or teeth commonly releases bacteria into the blood stream.

Animal experimentation seemed to provide evidence. Rosenow, by inoculating animals with a variety of strains of streptococci isolated from patients, believed he could demonstrate transmutation — changes in character, assumed virulence, and nature of the streptococci, some even becoming pneumococci, the bacteria which are the usual cause of lobar pneumonia. Strains of bacteria taken from human foci were grown, and these, when injected intravenously into animals, were claimed to produce specific damage to the heart, kidney, muscles or joints, comparable to the disease manifested by the patient. In addition, Rosenow and many other workers cultured bacteria from normally sterile parts of the bodies — stomach ulcers, joints, and muscle.

The fact that most people with low-grade infections of the teeth, sinuses, tonsils, and prostate were free of symptoms and enjoyed apparent good health was explained by wide variations in resistance or immunity to disease. It was further postulated that the resistance of the body to infection was decreased under the stress of exposure to cold, debility from physical and mental overwork, starvation. This supposition seemed plausible, though admittedly vague.

The theory postulated that many chronic diseases were due to the existence of foci or localized nests of bacteria of low virulence. These or their toxins entered the bloodstream from time to time and affected or invaded other parts of the body. These chronic infections were assumed to produce the disease of the system. William Hunter addressed the medical students at McGill University in 1910 with these heady words: "The worst cases of anemia, gastritis, colitis, of all kinds and degrees, of obscure fever of unknown origin, or purpura, or nervous disturbances of all kinds ranging from mental depression up to actual lesions of the cord, or chronic rheumatic affections, of kidney disease, are those which owe their origin to or are gravely complicated by oral sepsis [infection of the mouth]."

Billings and his group expanded the list of possible foci to include the entire gastrointestinal tract; the genital tract (vagina, uterus, prostate); the urinary tract (bladder, ureters, kidneys); as well as the teeth, mouth, tonsils and sinuses, which were already implicated.

The concept attracted far more advocates and enthusiasts than that of autointoxication, becoming highly respectable in medical circles and widely accepted. Indeed, it took advantage of the theories of autointoxication. As a result, a substantial segment of the population of North America and Great Britain (the physicians on the European continent were less gullible), was subjected to many forms of surgical and medical treatment. The surgery included.

1. *Extraction of teeth.* At first this was often limited to those obviously infected, but later it became customary to extract all the teeth in certain diseases, particularly in patients with arthritis.

2. *Tonsillectomy and adenoidectomy.* This became an extremely common procedure, particularly for those who could afford it. Some doctors argued that the large cryptic tonsils were abnormal or harboured organisms responsible for disease elsewhere. Others claimed that small firm ones were more likely the culprits. (Today it is admitted that it is impossible to tell by examination that tonsils are not infected, and it is known that about one in five healthy, normal school children harbours hemolytic streptococci in his throat.) Not only were tonsils extracted from patients with chronic disease such as arthritis, they were also removed from children to prevent colds and to guard against general ill health. Parents were made to feel neglectful if their children were allowed to grow up with both tonsils in place.

3. *Appendectomy.* Performed on a large scale for "chronic appendicitis," as in patients thought to have autointoxication. In addition, the appendix was commonly removed on suspicion that it might be the source of the chronic disease

troubling the patient. Many physicians routinely removed teeth, tonsils, and appendices from their arthritis patients.

4. *Removal of the gall bladder.* This became a common surgical procedure whenever the gall bladder was suspected of being the source of trouble.

5. *Excision of the uterus, the Fallopian tubes, or the ovaries.* Performed frequently if there was any indication either by bacterial culture or by the existence of lower abdominal tenderness that they might be foci.

6. *Prostatic surgery.* Not uncommon if prostatic massage produced evidence of low-grade infection.

7. *Lane's operation for removal of the colon.* Less common but not unusual. It was condemned by most conservative medical advocates of the theory.

Among the few advantages of the surgical treatment was a considerable improvement of the dental hygiene and diets of the patients. Teeth definitely decayed or abscessed were removed, often improving the patient's health. Some patients were helped by removal of grossly enlarged tonsils and obstructing adenoids, or truly infected gall bladders, or appendices.

In addition to these surgical procedures, a number of medical treatments were instituted for the host of diseases implicated. These included chronic application of antibacterial agents to the throat and sinuses (the silver compounds were commonly used), colonic irrigations, and prostatic massage. A variety of vaccines was prepared and injected into the patients. Some of the vaccines were made from killed bacteria isolated from the foci within the patient, called autogenous vaccines (here there is an obvious overlap with vaccine therapy of Almoth Wright); some were from mixtures of bacteria, usually strains of streptococci, the polyvalent vaccines.

Many of those treated were relieved at least temporarily of their symptoms and improved. This was particularly true of those with arthritis, nephritis, and rheumatic fever, diseases characterized by spontaneous cure or improvement in a large proportion of cases. Nearly all early articles advocating the theory were accompanied by a series of glowing anecdotal case reports of the improvement, or cures resulting from excision surgery.

Within a few years, the excesses, medical and surgical, resulting from the theory of focal infection appalled even its originators. Billings himself warned against "unnecessary" extraction of teeth, tonsils, and colons, and urged the preventive measures of proper diet, good hygiene, fresh air, appropriate rest and exercise, and even alternating hot and cold daily showers. Gradually a reaction set in. By the 1930s, evidence had accumulated that the concept was basically wrong. Initial enthusiasts, such as the influential Russel Cecil, professor of medicine at Cornell and editor of the standard textbook of medicine, reversed themselves. In 1933 Cecil wrote, "The keystone of modern treatment of rheumatoid arthritis is the elimination of infected foci." In 1938 he condemned the concept, which he felt was "reaching the status of an accepted fact." He did add, however, that he still believed the streptococcus to be implicated in rheumatoid arthritis.

The evidence refuting the theory was based on the failure to confirm the experiments and conclusions of Rosenow, and the observations of critical observers that patients were not benefited by the treatments. Other bacteriologists, re-examining Rosenow's data and repeating his experiments, found flaws in his techniques and could not demonstrate the selective affinity of bacteria for specific organs and tissues, claimed by Rosenow. The green streptococcus of low virulence so often said to be the source of trouble could not be shown to have a causal relationship to any systemic disease other than subacute bacterial endocarditis.

Comparisons of the results of treatment were made in several large series of arthritic patients (300 to 500 cases). Those who had had all or most of their teeth removed were no better than those who had not. (It was pointed out that about one-fourth of the patients with rheumatoid arthritis recover, one-half improve, and one-fourth get worse, no matter what the treatment. The results today are better.)

Analyses of series of children failed to demonstrate the benefit of tonsillectomy. A British commission investigated 30,000 school children and found that the incidence of colds, coughs, and sore throats did not differ between those with or those without their tonsils. About one-half of the group had had their tonsils removed. The commission concluded, ". . . there is a tendency for the operation to be performed as a routine, prophylactic ritual for no particular reason and with no particular result."

Furthermore, it was recognized that many patients were being harmed. Though rare, deaths, lung abscesses and bacterial endocarditis occurred as a result of some of the tonsillectomies and tooth extractions. Between 1931 and 1935 in England, 513 deaths were reported as being due to tonsillectomy.

By the forties, there was general agreement (with rare exceptions) on the part of most teachers of medicine that the results had been a therapeutic nightmare. In contrast with the theories of autointoxication and its treatment, no Molière or Shaw pilloried the absurdities and advocates of foci of infection. Within the profession, however, there was bitterness. An Austrian internist, Verhoeff, stated, "Belief in focal infection must be taken, like religion, on faith." A pathologist commented wryly that a focus was anything which could be removed surgically.

In 1949 the *Primer on Rheumatic Disease,* prepared by the American Rheumatism Association, issued the warning, "No one now believes that the removal of an infected focus will alter the course of rheumatoid arthritis, and extraction of teeth, tonsils, gallbladders, and pelvic organs is to be condemned unless they are so diseased that they should be removed for their own sakes. Indeed, wholesale removal of teeth is not only useless but actually harmful to the patient through interference with nutrition."

Yet, four years later, in *Comroes' Arthritis,* Graham complained that, "Despite a complete absence of controlled observations pointing to its validity, the theory of focal infections still ranks first in the minds of many physicians and dentists when confronted with a rheumatic patient. In many instances the removal of teeth and tonsils is not only the first but the only treatment recommended."

Even now in the 1970s tonsils continue to be extracted more often than necessary. Non-specific or autogenous vaccines of no proven value are still sold and used.

X-Ray Treatment to the Thymus of Infants

As early as 1614 and subsequently during the following centuries, the death of an infant was ascribed by physicians to suffocation due to pressure from an enlarged thymus; the soft gland, shaped like the leaf of the thyme plant, located in the upper chest just in front of the trachea and the large arteries which arise from the heart and immediately below the thyroid gland. Inasmuch as the thymus is normally large during early infancy, and sudden unexplained death — often called crib or cot death — is an occasional occurrence at this age, the connection was plausible.

However, in 1889 Paltauf, an Austrian pathologist, formulated a somewhat different explanation for unaccountable sudden deaths. He observed that, at autopsy, the thymus and lymphatic tissues frequently appeared enlarged in persons of all ages who died suddenly from unknown or trivial causes, and argued that the deaths were due to a general condition which he termed *status thymicolymphaticus*. The explanation was accepted by many physicians. Since the function of the thymus was totally unknown at that time and remained so until the 1960s, it was a difficult idea to disprove. (The thymus is now known to be essential for the cellular immune responses which protect against certain infections and possibly cancerous cells as well. It also is concerned with the responses to transfusions and transplants.)

In 1907 Friedlander, an American pediatrician, reported successful treatment by x-irradiation of a seriously ill infant with breathing difficulty. The thymus had appeared much enlarged in the diagnostic x-ray film. Films taken after irradiation of the neck and chest of the patient showed the thymus gland to be much smaller. The baby recovered and thrived. This simple, apparently harmless treatment, advocated soon thereafter by some leading pediatricians, became popular in the United States and Canada. In the American press, stories of babies being saved from "thymic death" became common. Acceptance of the treatment was limited in England; few Continental doctors resorted to it. Between 1910 and 1950, many thousands of infants were irradiated. There was no question that following irradiation the thymus almost invariably became smaller — such x-ray treatment will shrink almost any thymus — and most of the distressed infants recovered. In some hospitals it became customary to make a diagnostic x-ray of the chest of every newborn. If the thymus was found to be large treatment with irradiation was carried out as a preventive measure.

In the meantime, the concept of *status thymicolymphaticus* was gradually being disproved. A series of investigations showed that there were wide variations in the size of the human thymus in persons dying suddenly from well-defined causes, such as accidents, strokes, heart attacks. The normal range in thymic size was proven to be unusually great in young infants, and the thymus was found to be normally largest in relation to body weight at birth. Edith Potter, the American pathologist and a recognized authority on the fetus and the newborn, wrote in 1953 that she had never seen evidence of compression of the trachea or other ill effects of thymic enlargement. Additionally, observant pediatricians noted that many young infants with respiratory distress recover spontaneously without treatment. No controlled studies of treated and untreated patients were ever performed.

In 1950 Duffy and Fitzgerald, two investigators at the Sloan-Kettering Cancer Institute in New York, reported ten cases of cancer of the thyroid gland in adolescent children who had been irradiated during infancy. Only a few cases of cancer of this type at this age had been previously reported; the finding of a cluster of such cases made the association between irradiation and cancer seem suspicious. As early as 1902 cancer had been reported in man as a result of exposure to ionizing radiation, but the physicians treating infants did not believe that the small x-ray doses used could be harmful.

Subsequently it was reported that among all instances of cancer of the thyroid occurring in young people in the United States a majority had a history of x-ray treatment during infancy or early childhood. Winship and Rosvoll collected 704 cases of this form of cancer by amassing reports from the world medical literature and by corresponding with hospitals in twenty-seven countries. Two facts were evident: 1. There had been a sharp increase in the number of such cases beginning in 1940, and a decrease from 1960 on; 2. Whenever the information was available there was a history of x-ray treatment of the thymus in 80 per cent of the cases from the United States. (Others had received x-ray or radium treatments to shrink the tonsils or adenoids.)

Proof that the association between the x-ray therapy and the cancer occurring when the patients were in their teens or twenties was not due to chance was provided by Simpson and her co-workers in 1955. They found thirteen cases of cancer among 1,400 children who had been exposed to this treatment as infants. No cases had occurred among the 1,795 untreated siblings. In 1967 Hemplemann, a radiologist in Rochester, New York, reported a long-term follow-up study on 3,000 persons treated with x-rays in infancy for alleged enlargement of the thymus. Most of the tumours which had occurred were in a group of 500 who had received x-ray administered to the front and back of the chest. He concluded, "The increase in the numbers of cases of thyroid cancer over that expected to occur in a comparable group of non-irradiated individuals was 233 times the expectation for persons treated." The dose of x-ray did not relate to the probability that the patient would develop cancer, though concentration of x-rays did. The age at irradiation did not affect the time in life when the cancer developed. (Some patients received treatment in childhood.) Almost all cases occurred during the patients' teens and twenties. To explain these findings, Hempleman hypothesized that the radiation damaged the chromosomes of the thyroid cells, and the rapid hormonal change occurring during adolescence caused some of the cells with the injured chromosomes to become cancerous. A similar situation appears to exist with respect to the association between stilbestrol given during pregnancy and the occurrence of vaginal cancer in the daughters born of such pregnancies (See Chapter 3).

Finally, it has been possible to produce cancer in rats by comparable doses of x-ray which do not impair the function of the thyroid gland.

While it is not proven beyond doubt, there is a very strong statistical probability of a causal relationship. It seems clear that x-irradiation of the thymus based on the erroneous concept of *status thymicolyphaticus* was not beneficial, and, in addition, was responsible for cancer of the thyroid in several hundred persons. The procedure has been abandoned as a serious hazard.

A New Blood Supply to the Heart Muscle

Two operations were based on the concept of revascularization — the creation of a new blood supply to a tissue or organ. In the first instance, the organ was the heart; in the second, the brain. Both surgical procedures were ineffective because of poor understanding of anatomy and physiology.

Just prior to the First World War, it had been recognized that an inadequate blood supply to the heart muscle itself (an insufficient blood flow through the coronary arteries) is a major cause of death. This is almost always due to the effects of arteriosclerosis — narrowing or plugging of the coronary arteries which directly supply the heart. Beginning in 1936 a series of operations was devised aimed at improving the coronary circulation by providing it with artificial intercommunicating additional circulation. Adhesions were artificially produced between the surface of the heart and other tissue: flaps of muscle from the chest wall; the omentum (the apron-like fold of peritoneum in the abdomen); the pericardium (the fibrous sac which surrounds the heart). These adhesions were made by direct suture, or, in the case of the pericardium, by introducing an irritating substance such as talc into the pericardial sac. Blood vessels grew into these adhesions. The initial results were reported as good, particularly by the respective surgeons who originated the operations. Many patients were relieved of the attacks of the crushing chest pains of angina pectoris, which characterizes an inadequate coronary circulation. No controlled studies were made at that time of these procedures, and their true value remains undetermined. (In recent years, these techniques have been replaced by other operations which directly increase the blood supply to the heart by removing or by-passing with vein or arterial grafts the arteriosclerotic obstructions.) All of the early procedures required opening the chest, and carried a significant risk, the fatality rates being 5 to 10 per cent.

For many years, anatomists had been able to demonstrate, by injection of coloured dyes or particles, natural inter-communicating arterial channels between the small branches of the coronary arteries and the vessels of other organs. It had been shown that these connections were stimulated to grow and develop in dogs, by narrowing or obstructing the dog's coronary arteries. This was particularly true of intercommunications between the coronary circulation and the network of arteries arising from the first branches of the two internal "mammary" arteries. These vessels lie just inside the wall of the chest in front of the base of the heart and are easily accessible through simple small incisions made between the first two ribs alongside the breast bone. The chest need not be opened. In 1939 an Italian surgeon reasoned that ligation (tying off) of the two internal mammary arteries just beyond the branches which connected with the heart muscle would increase the blood supply to the heart by increasing the pressure in these branches, thereby forcing more blood to flow through the intercommunicating small arteries. He operated on one patient suffering from intractible angina pectoris. Two years later the patient was living and comfortable. In spite of this good result, the operation was not done again until the 1950s, when it was revived by a group of Italian surgeons who reported (in 1955) on seventy cases, sixty-four of them alive and improved. Upon learning of these results, a well-known group of cardiac surgeons in Philadelphia enthusiastically took up the procedure, after proving on dogs to their own satisfaction that the operation increased the blood pressure in the first branches of the internal mammary arteries behind the ligatures and the flow of blood through the inter-communication into the heart muscle. In a small series of dogs with appropriate comparison controls, they showed that, after tying off one of the major coronary arteries, more of the animals with ligated internal mammary arteries survived. They then quickly embarked on a large uncontrolled series of operations on persons seriously incapacitated by inadequate coronary circulation, most of whom suffered from angina pectoris. Within a year and a half, they had performed the surgery on 150 patients, about two-thirds of whom were entirely free of pain or were much improved during the early months after the operations.

The procedure was relatively simple; the surgical fatality low — less than one per cent; the results seemed to be good; and the disease was common. Surgeons in Italy and the United States enthusiastically adopted the technique, and in three years many hundreds of operations were done, of which 456 were reported in medical journals. Other observers confirmed the favourable results. Not only did most of the patients feel better, but they could carry on ordinary activities. In some instances, the surgery was followed by changes toward normal in the electrocardiogram.

However, skepticism regarding the value of the procedure remained in the minds of many physicians. Sabiston and Blalock, two outstanding cardiac surgeons at Johns Hopkins, performed a series of experiments on dogs, designed 1) to measure the amount of blood flowing through the small channels between the first branch of the internal mammary artery and the coronary circulation, before and after ligation of the internal mammary artery; and 2) to study the value of the procedure in protecting the animal subjected to ligation of a major coronary artery. Their techniques were meticulous and well planned. They concluded, ". . . the volume of blood flowing through the internal mammary artery following ligation in the second intercostal space is quite small . . . the procedure does not protect against experimental coronary occlusion."

The conclusive evidence which discredited this attempt to revascularize the heart came from two carefully controlled clinical trials using a sham operation — a surgical placebo — for one-half of the patients chosen at random. The plans were explained to the participants in advance. A double-blind technique was used. Half the patients had the internal mammary arteries exposed and ligated; the other half had them simply exposed but not ligated. A total of only thirty-five patients took part, fourteen had skin incisions only. Of these fourteen, ten patients were much better; their pain disappeared, and their exercise tolerance improved. Several were able to return to work. A few showed evidence of improvement in the electrocardiogram. Such was the strong psychologic effect of the incision alone. The results were equally good in those who had undergone the genuine operation, with ligation of both internal mammary arteries. Unfortunately, in neither group did the beneficial results last.

As a result of this trial on a small number of patients, an operation which had been enthusiastically accepted in the United States was abandoned within two years after it was introduced. Not only was it discredited, but, in addition, physicians were made skeptical of the claims of future surgery for angina pectoris. Thousands of persons were saved from undergoing unnecessary surgery.

A New Blood Supply to the Brain

The approach to the creation of a new blood supply to the brain was entirely different. In 1949 three physicians at the Western Reserve University Medical School in Cleveland introduced a new operative procedure designed to increase the arterial blood supply to the cortex of the brain for some patients with mental retardation, cerebral palsy and convulsions. The operation consisted in directly connecting, side-to-side, the large carotid artery on the right side of the neck and the internal jugular vein, and of ligating the vein just below the connection so that blood would no longer drain through it back into the heart. The high pressure in the artery forced the oxygenated arterial blood through the connection, and, in a reverse direction up the jugular vein into the veins of the brain. It was assumed that this arterial blood would be forced also into the capillaries, thereby providing increased oxygen to nerve cells. The second assumption was that, in patients suffering from damage to the brain resulting in mental retardation, convulsions, and cerebral palsy, there are many surviving but non-functioning nerve cells present which could be revived by increasing their blood supply in this fashion. The surgery was relatively simple and appeared to carry a low risk. The initial results on 125 patients, most of whom were children, were encouraging. About a third of the children were more alert, had improved general behaviour, higher I.Q. scores, decreased spasticity. Convulsions disappeared for weeks or months. Glowing reports of individual successes were cited in the press, causing desperate parents of retarded or spastic children to travel to Cleveland from all over the United States.

Because the surgery was technically simple and the need great, other surgeons in the United States, France, Sweden and Norway began performing the operation. Three hundred and fifty-six were reported in the next four years, and it is probable that many more operations were done but not reported. The later results failed to confirm the early successes. It is true that many unfortunate parents who had expected much from the procedure declared that their children were brighter, more alert, better behaved, and less unstable. It was true also that the hospitalized child was given special attention and care. More critical evaluation of the intelligence tests showed that the changes in I.Q. of those who improved were not sufficient to be considered significant. Seizures returned after a few months.

The early experience of few complications and absence of fatality was not borne out. Up to six per cent of the patients died during or shortly after surgery; some became worse, with more convulsions and increased mental retardation; a few sustained heart failure. Further investigations clearly revealed that while the arterial blood did reach the veins on the surface of the brain, it did not enter the capillaries. It was shunted off into many other interconnecting veins on the left side. The entire concept appears to have been basically erroneous and ill-conceived. Within four years of its introduction, the operation was abandoned by general consent.

Russel Meyers, chief of neurosurgery at the University of Iowa, in 1958 expressed the opinion shared by many surgeons: "Demonstration of its clinical ineptitude has by now been sufficiently adduced to warrant its being discarded. Progress in medicine is, of course, made by just such disclosures. The lamentable thing is that we seldom arrive at such conclusive answers within so short a period of time as here exemplified."

Gluing of Fractures

Another abandoned surgical method of treatment which now also appears to have been due to an error of concept was that of attempting to glue together fractured bones in the 1950s.

It is said that the ancient Egyptians made a counterpart of the modern plaster cast for fractures by impregnating bandages with pitch resins, and that Hippocrates records the use of splints, both systems designed for the immobilization of limbs. But not until this century were successful attempts made to directly fasten the broken ends of exposed bones together. Sir Arbuthnot Lane was one of the pioneers in the use of various types of metal screws, pins, and plates, many of which are still in use. With the explosive development of plastics following the Second World War, the use of tissue adhesives or "glue" became a medical dream. Its application to fractures would permit the patient to return to normal activity sooner — perhaps in a day or so — and foreign material need not remain in the body. In a review in 1964 Dr. Karl-Axel Rietz, a Swedish surgeon at the Karolinska Institute, summarized the requirements: "Such bonding agents should be nontoxic, innocuous to tissue and should not retard healing of bone. They should in time be excreted from the body and, of course, must be free of carcinogenic properties."

The first report of success came from the Soviet Union. G. V. Golovin in 1956, in an article entitled (in translation), "The Possibility to Stick Together Bone Fractures," told of his experimental use of epoxy resins — adhesives widely used commercially in moulding and gluing because of their great strength, adhesives, and resistance to corrosion. A hardener or curing agent is added to pastelike resin and applied to the surfaces involved and allowed to set for a matter of hours.

Two years after the Russian report and without knowledge of it, an Australian orthopedic surgeon, Bernard Bloch, wrote in Sydney a personal account in the *Journal of Bone and Joint Surgery,* which began: "Two years ago I began experimental research into the bonding of fractures by amine-cured ethoxyline resins which are used in industry as adhesives. The first experiments were carried out on the forelegs of sheep. The results of these were so encouraging that in 1958, the technique was applied to fractures in humans." After testing for toxicity and sterility, Bloch tried his technique on thirty-one sheep, with success in twenty-one (three became infected). Then he applied his approach, with gratifying success, to two patients whose badly fractured bones had failed to unite after the use of conventional splints and bone plates.

That same year, an orthopedist from Philadelphia, Michael Mandarino, presented to a meeting of the American Association for the Surgery of Trauma a case which attracted the attention of surgeons from many countries. An oblique fracture of the tibia had been glued with a plastic, Ostamer; three days later the patient was walking about without a cast or crutches. During the next three years, Mandarino and his colleague, Salvator, published a series of reports of the experiments and their success using this entirely different substance, polyurethane foam plastic. The technique consisted of exposure and cleaning of the broken ends of bone, preparation of a trough along it, and removal of fat and moisture from the central canal. The plastic, to which a hardening catalyst and a foaming agent were added, was then poured into it. In about half an hour it hardened into a firm mass which filled the central canal of the bone; the excess plastic was removed. The two surgeons believed that the new bone grew into the plastic. Initially there was some enthusiasm for this approach, both in the United States and in Italy. By June 1959 Mandarino and Salvatore were able to collect reports of 220 cases treated with Ostamer; 93 per cent of these had been successful. They attributed the failures to technical errors. Fractures of the femur, the humerus, sternum, hip, tibia, spine, and the knee joint were said to have been treated successfully by this method, termed "osteosynthesis."

Also in 1959 the Russian Golovin published enthusiastic follow-up reports on 32 human subjects — all successful. Thereafter he seems to have written no more on the subject.

Then, in the 1960s, reports from other surgeons began to appear, with accounts of failures and serious complications. In one series of 51 operations, there were only nine successes. Breakage of the glue and its failure to adhere to the bone seemed to be the problem. In addition, chronic wound infections were common complications, the plastic foam appearing to act as an irritant foreign body, retarding the healing of bone.

Mandarino and Salvatore continued animal experiments to prove that Ostamer was not toxic and was a strong binder of bone. They performed 110 operations on 66 dogs, bonding the broken ends of femurs and radii, and came to the conclusion that the plastic dissolved slowly, permitting the bone to grow through the defect in four-fifths of the cases. However, accumulated experience from many other animal experiments in various countries indicated that the plastic retarded healing, that it did not dissolve, that new bone did not grow through it, and that it tended to act as an irritant foreign body. One worker found that break-down products of polyurethane plastic can have carcinogenic action in animals.

The error in concept appears to have been the hypothesis that the plastic would 1) gradually dissolve, being replaced by bone, and 2) that it would stimulate bone growth. In fact, it appeared to prevent the periosteum — the thin layer of growing cells on the surface of the bone — from participating in new bone growth. The plastics and resins did act successfully as splints in many cases, though they were not as strong as the metal plate and rods then in use.

No controlled clinical study was made. The approach was given up chiefly because the long-range results were so disappointing, often disastrous. As one author stated, "glue" became a medical bad word. Now it is apparent that the adhesives were used in man prematurely without adequate animal trials and investigation.

Insulin Coma Treatment of Schizophrenia

Insulin coma therapy of schizophrenia was a treatment almost universally used for a quarter of a century and gradually given up, in part because of adverse reactions, in part because of the demonstration of its ineffectiveness in controlled clinical trials, and in part because of the appearance of the highly effective new psychotropic drugs.

Severe mental diseases without known cause have always been one of Man's major problems. Until the fifties, schizophrenia accounted for more than half the inmates in mental hospitals, a major cause of disability affecting at one time or another a significant percentage of the population. The term, which means literally "mind splitting," is descriptive of the characteristic loss of contact with reality, the delusions and hallucinations, the bizarre behaviour, the private fantasies manifested by the unfortunate victims of this disease. Don Quixote, the hero of Cervantes' novel, has been thought to be a classic example. Because of much fragmentary evidence, schizophrenia is now suspected of being a genetically determined biochemical abnormality. But it is still not known whether it is basically a single disease with many manifestations or a group of related diseases. Its course is highly variable and unpredictable, with frequent remissions and recurrences, occasional spontaneous recoveries, and common progressive deterioration, making evaluation of any treatment difficult. Moreover, there are no specific laboratory tests with which to establish the diagnosis.

Until the 1930s there was little to offer other than custodial care, and patients were often committed to mental instiutions for life. Electric shock therapy, dramatic and hazardous, devised early in the decades, seemed clearly to offer temporary help to many afflicted. In 1933 Manfred Sakel, a young neuro-psychiatrist in Berlin, reported his results employing insulin coma therapy which is equally drastic and more dangerous. In treating diabetes with the hormone insulin, which became available in 1923, it was found that an excess produced the feared complications of coma and often convulsions. The treatment of schizophrenia was the result of Sakel's observation that the accidental overdose of insulin given to a diabetic morphine addict appeared to clear up the addict's confused mental state. He hypothesized that in schizophrenia, distorted, unhealthy, abnormal pathways occurred between the nerve cells, replacing the normal connections. He believed insulin, by forcing sugar out of the blood and into the cells, produced a temporary blockade of all metabolic activity or "hibernation" of nerve cells, disrupting sick and defective pathways and allowing restoration of dormant, healthy, pre-existing connections. Repeated treatments were required in order to completely destroy the abnormal connections. It seemed apparent that many psychotic patients were improved — at least temporarily. Sakel was enthusiastic about his results. Many reported studies by others supported his claims, and for more than twenty years the use of insulin coma was universally accepted in the treatment of schizophenia. It introduced the era of biological treatment of psychoses and served to cause these diseases to be reparded as physiological problems which could be treated by drugs and other methods, just as other illnesses were.

After the initial enthusiasm, a reaction gradually set in as the years went by. Insulin in the large doses used causes sweating, rapid, sometimes irregular, heart action, anxiety, abdominal discomfort, and sometimes vomiting, before the patient loses consciousness. Rare deaths and instances of serious irreversible brain damage were reported. The treatments required intensive medical and nursing supervision in order to minimize the adverse reactions. Gradually, many physicians became skeptical of the benefits. A number of workers compared insulin-treated patients with parallel control groups cared for under the same general condition; the results were variable, most indicating little or no difference between the two groups. However, there was no well-planned clinical trial until 1957 when three English psychiatrists, Ackner, Harris and Oldham, reported a reassessment of insulin coma, arguing that if it were ineffective, it should be abandoned; that if it were of value, it should not be entirely given up in favour of the recently introduced drug chlorpromazine. Their trial was well conceived. Each patient in the control group was carefully matched with a patient in the treated group for age, sex, subtype of the disease, and duration of symptoms. Patients were randomly selected and treated at the same time and under general conditions. In addition, a double-blind approach was used. The patient and the physicians evaluating the results were carefully kept unaware of the identity of those who had received insulin. All patients were told they were having "coma" treatment. Deep sleep was induced with barbiturates in the control group. All patients received the same number of injections and doses of medicine during the day. Though only fifty patients (twenty-five matched pairs) were involved, the results were so clear-cut as to be obvious without statistical analyses. Of the control patients, ten were symptom-free and apparently fully recovered, four had some residual defect, and eleven were still psychotic. Of the patients treated with insulin, nine were fully recovered, four had residual defect, and eleven were still psychotic. (One of the insulin-treated patients was killed while bicycling after discharge from the hospital.) In 1962 Ackner and Oldham reported on the three-year follow-up of their initial study. The findings confirmed the initial results — that the insulin did not seem to have a specific effect. It now seems probable that the intense care and attention required by the patients undergoing repeated episodes of insulin coma probably accounted for many of the apparently beneficial results. It is still true today that insulin has no proven pharmacological action in schizophrenia.

These results so strongly indicated that insulin was not of specific value that they were influential in inducing many psychiatrists to abandon this difficult and dangerous form of treatment. It was completely given up in most western nations only as it was replaced by the new, highly effective psychotropic drugs. Chlorpromazine, the first and still the most effective of these in the treatment of schizophrenia, was introduced in 1952 by Jean Delay, a French psychiatrist, but it took almost eight years until its value as compared to that of a placebo was clearly and unmistakably established. This lag was due in part to the fact that in the initial controlled trials, the doses employed were too small. By 1972 there were ten chemical classes of compounds which had been shown to be effective in relieving the symptoms and favourably altering the course of the disease. As yet no cure is known.

These new drugs have radically changed the outlook for many of these patients. Now, with their use, aided by more intelligent and humane care and occasional electric convulsive therapy (ECT), the length of time required for hospitalization of patients for psychotic attacks is commonly a matter of weeks or months. Subsequent treatment — since most patients need to remain on medication — can be carried out with the patients living at home and attending clinics or doctors' offices. Thousands of people have been able to return to useful, enjoyable and active lives, one of the major accomplishments of twentieth-century medicine. The disease of Van Gogh and Nijinski has been brought under partial control.

Freezing of Stomachs

Another form of ineffective treatment given up because of the results of a careful double-blind controlled clinical study was the freezing of stomachs for treatment of peptic ulcer.

Though most people realize that an ulcer is any open sore, an inflamed raw area anywhere on the surface of the body or on the mucous mebrane lining parts within it, so common is the disease that the unspecified term is usually taken to indicate a peptic ulcer involving either the stomach or the duodenum (the first portion of the small intestine). Peptic ulcer is known to affect many millions — some have estimated twenty per cent of all adults in Europe and North America. The causes remain poorly understood; the treatment, less than satisfactory largely, trial and error. While most who are afflicted live with their disease, it remains a world-wide medical problem of major proportions.

Ulcer patients who fail to respond to medical and other measures may require surgical removal of part of the stomach — gastrectomy — for relief of their pain. Owen Wagensteen, professor of surgery at the University of Minnesota Medical School and known the world over for his important contributions to the problems of intestinal obstruction, gave the prestigious Moynihan lecture to the Royal College of Surgeons in London in January 1962. He discussed the history of the physiology of the stomach and proposed a new method of treatment of peptic ulcer — gastric freezing — which he believed could replace gastrectomy. In the spring of the same year he and his colleagues gave a more detailed but still preliminary report at the annual meeting of the American Medical Association. (Four years previously, Wagensteen and his co-workers had reported effective relief of gastric hemorrhage by local cooling of the stomach. The cooling for hemorrhage became a useful procedure.) The technique consisted of lowering the temperature of the stomach to approximately 0° Fahrenheit ($-18°$ Celsius) for an hour, by flushing cooled absolute alcohol in and out of a large balloon inserted into the stomach, the balloon connected to a refrigerating unit by a combined double tube allowing the alcohol to be circulated through it. The insertion of the balloon was through the patient's mouth, after anesthetizing his throat in order to minimize discomfort. Wagensteen and his co-workers had first experimented on 150 dogs, in order to determine the safety and effectiveness of the method. They learned that no permanent harm occurred to the lining of a dog's stomach after it had been frozen "hard as a rock" by this method for periods of more than an hour. They found that in both the dogs and in twenty-four patients with ulcers the freezing depressed the volume of gastric secretions and their acidity. The concept propounded inhibition of the gastric secretion to allow healing of ulcers.

All twenty-four of the patients experienced relief of their symptoms. The authors concluded their report; "It would appear that something akin to a physiological gastrectomy can be achieved by a temporary period of gastric freezing. When well controlled no harm results to the patient or to his stomach."[1] They added that if gastric secretions and symptoms returned, the treament could be repeated.

This was a dramatic and highly publicized procedure; it was relatively simple and seemed to work, and an outstanding group headed by an eminent surgeon announced its effectiveness. Gastric freezing machines for circulation of the coolant became a necessary piece of equipment for many hospitals and clinics in many countries.

A year and a half later, Wagensteen's group presented an interim follow-up report at the annual meeting of the American Medical Association. Their experience, together with that of five local hospitals and five other outside university clinics around the United States, totalled 841 patients, none of whom had died. About 7 per cent, however, had either bleeding or secondary ulcers, which seemed to have been produced by the freezing. Seventy per cent of Wagensteen's patients were free of symptoms initially, but only 50 per cent of them remained so for more than a year.

After the initial enthusiasm, reports began to appear of disappointing results and increasing complications, with rare deaths. Many became skeptical of the value of this approach. An editorial in the *Journal of the American Medical Association* suggested that, because of the conflicting reports of the value of gastric freezing, only a controlled study with patients selected at random, and careful statistical evaluation applied, could provide a definitive answer. Three limited studies were undertaken. Two were published in 1964; one in 1965. The first two of these involved approximately twenty patients in the freezing group and in the control group. The relief of pain was about the same initially in each group, but there was no substantial reduction of gastric secretion. At six months, the improvement was more noticeable in the frozen group in one study, but not in the other. In the third study, from Columbia University College of Physicians and Surgeons in New York, there were thirty patients in each group. Both groups demonstrated a good initial symptomatic response, but the frozen group maintained a statistically significant superiority for at least six months. Also, the frozen group experienced suppression of acid secretion lasting two months, in contrast to the control, in which there was none.

Because of the disagreement, the problem remained unsettled until a fourth study, initiated in 1963, was published in 1969. This was the result of careful planning and close co-operation of five institutions in the United States — four major medical schools and one large hospital. Eighty-two patients comprised the freeze group; 78 were subjects in a sham procedure. The techniques were identical in every way, except that tap water at body temperature was circulated through the balloons placed in the stomachs of the control group. The details are of some interest. Each institution was supplied with envelopes numbered serially to insure randomization. When the patient had been prepared and the balloon inserted, the envelope was opened. This contained a card indicating whether the coolant at − °C. or tap water at 37° (normal body temperature) was to be used. The biostatisticians controlling the study had arranged that there were no significant differences between the two groups with regard to age, duration of ulcers (average nine years), history of previous bleeding from ulcer, severity of pain, classification of moderate or severe symptoms, or x-ray changes. Neither the patient nor the examining physicians were aware of the nature of the treatment until the end of the study two years later. All patients were admitted to the hospital and evaluated on the basis of clinical history, physical examination, analysis of gastric secretion, upper gastrointestinal x-rays at six weeks, and at three, six, twelve, eighteen and twenty-four months after the procedure. At six weeks, 29 per cent of the patients in both groups relapsed.

At no time was there a significant difference in those who underwent a sham procedure and those who were frozen. The same was true with respect to gastric secretions.

The authors summarized as follows: "The results of this study demonstrate conclusively that the freezing procedure was no better than the sham in the treatment of duodenal ulcer."

An additional independent investigation on animals provided more evidence. Experimental studies of the procedure in dogs and pigs showed that the actual freezing of the wall of the stomach occurred erratically and unpredictably, involving variable areas rather than the whole organ. Whatever portions of the stomach were truly frozen developed dead tissue. In other words, it seemed that Wagensteen's concept of suppressing gastric secretions and acidity by temporarily injuring tissue did not hold.

As a result of all these studies, the technique was given up within a few years after its introduction. Though rare, there were serious complications. The claimed benefits were not proven.

CHAPTER TWO

Laboratory Mistakes and Accidents

The preparation of vaccines for the prevention of infective disease has been beset with problems since the days of Pasteur. By and large, serious toxic effects have been limited to relatively small numbers of patients, in spite of the fact that millions have been vaccinated. However, three tragic large-scale incidents called attention to the extreme care required in the preparation of these preventative biological agents: tuberculosis and death in infants and children caused by the administration of a virulent strain of the bacillus, rather than the live attenuated vaccine called BCG (the Lübeck disaster); vaccination of children, with inadequately killed poliomyelitis virus, causing paralytic polio in children (the Cutter incident); and the production of hepatitis on a large scale in soldiers vaccinated during the Second World War with yellow fever vaccine contaminated by the hepatitis virus. Three other episodes involved useful synthetic drugs. In each instance the tragedy was caused by mistakes or accidents in the laboratory.

The basic medications — BCG, killed polio vaccine, yellow fever vaccine, potassium chloride, sulfanilamide, and hexachlorophene — are effective agents in the prevention or treatment of disease. In contrast to most of the errors analyzed in the other sections, these mistakes were quickly recognized and rectified.

Lübeck Disaster — BCG

Between 1891 and 1930, a series of minor calamities occurred as a result of immunization of patients in the attempt to prevent various diseases, including diphtheria, cholera, typhoid fever, and tuberculosis.

In addition to hepatitis with jaundice following the vaccinations for smallpox occurring in 1890 (Chapter 6), there were a small number of cases of tetanus following vaccines given for cholera in 1902, and a few deaths after administration of diphtheria antitoxin in 1924. But the first large, serious epidemic attracting worldwide attention was the Lübeck disaster in 1930 in Germany, as a result of the administration to infants of virulent tubercle bacilli, rather than BCG.

During the nineteenth and twentieth centuries, tuberculosis was the "white plague" most threatening the civilized world — the captain of the men of death. It carried off more young men and women than did any other disease, and influenced literature from Abbé Prévost's *Manon Lescaut* to Thomas Mann's *Magic Mountain*. The dying tubercular heroine was a standard figure. Robert Koch's demonstration in 1882 of the specific agent — the tubercle bacillus — which caused tuberculosis, resulted in a rush of efforts to produce a vaccine for the prevention of the disease. Koch himself had introduced a tuberculin vaccine for *treatment,* with disastrous results. The most fruitful efforts were those of Calmette, one of the outstanding French bacteriologists, and his associate, Guérin. Between 1907 and 1921, the two men worked at preparing a safe and effective vaccine. Their experiments on cattle led them to the conclusion that immunity could result only from infection by a living organism. They therefore prepared a vaccine by attenuating the virulence of living bovine tubercle bacilli, much as Sabin was to do later with the poliomyelitis virus. They subcultured seventy successive generations over a three-year period on a medium of potato, glycerine, and bile salts, until a massive dose of these living bacteria grown for years outside the body could be tolerated by calves. The calves were followed several years to make certain they did not develop the disease. Because of the bacteriologists' intense concern for the safety of this living vaccine — they were afraid it might regain its previous virulence — they tested it extensively on animals including monkeys. Since Calmette believed that prevention should begin at birth, he made careful trials on newborn infants between 1921 and 1924. These were followed by mass production of the vaccine now called *Bacille-Calmette-Guérin,* or BCG, in the Pasteur Institute. At the same time, strains were made available to foreign countries. Four hundred thousand infants were given the vaccine without deleterious effects.

Unfortunately, Calmette and Guérin did not use the same critical care in assessing the effectiveness of the vaccine that they had employed in insuring its safety. Their statistics comparing large numbers of vaccinated and unvaccinated children were severely criticized. They compared mortality data from all causes, not tuberculosis alone; they made obvious careless errors in arithmetic; there was no real controlled trial, even of the type recognized at that time. The skepticism regarding their data was in part responsible for the delay in acceptance of BCG as an effective and safe preventative.

The other problem related to the persistent concern of other bacteriologists that BCG might regain its virulence and become dangerous. In the spring of 1930 this was thought to have occurred in Lübeck, Germany. Two hundred and fifty-one newborn babies were given "BCG" by mouth; 207 developed clinical tuberculosis; of these, 72 died and 135 eventually recovered. There was worldwide coverage in the press of this disaster, and an official investigation followed. As a result, two doctors were sent to prison for their carelessness.

The inquiry and trial lasted until 1932. The official conclusion was that BCG had not reverted to its virulent state. Rather, the disaster had resulted from careless substitution of the vaccine with highly virulent human tubercle bacilli. Nevertheless, in the minds of many, BCG was considered dangerous, and its general acceptance was delayed. The use of BCG in France and the Scandinavian countries continued, but it was not until after the Second World War that it became widely used in Britain and the United States. Twenty-five years later, large-scale critical controlled studies with careful statistical analyses did establish that BCG produced a fourfold reduction in the hazard of contracting tuberculosis following exposure, thereby saving thousands of lives throughout the world.

Diethylene Glycol — "Elixir of Sulfanilamide"

Quite a different type of laboratory mistake — that of omission — was made with sufanilamide.

The era of chemotherapy against micro-organisms had been initiated by Ehrlich in 1906, with the use of salvarsan against the spirochaeta of syphilis, yaws, and relapsing fever. But in spite of persistent efforts, many years passed before effective antibacterial agents were discovered. Then in 1932 Domagk, a German pharmacologist, demonstrated the effectiveness of synthetic red dye prontosil in treating streptococcal and staphylococcal infecions in mice, and the pharmaceutical revolution began. Large-scale tests on animals confirmed the value and safety of the drug. It was then used cautiously on patients with the usually fatal streptococcic septicemia, then called "blood poisoning" by the laity. One of the first patients to be successfully treated was Domagk's daughter. Shortly thereafter, the Pasteur Institute of Paris isolated the active molecule in prontosil — the synthetic chemical sufanilamide. Because of their effectiveness in many previously hopeless diseases, the sulfonamide compounds were hailed by the newspapers as the "miracle drugs." The whole outlook of the treatment of an array of infectious diseases changed.

Sulfanilamide came into general use in the United States in 1937 and was marketed under many trade names. In the fall of that year in the United States, a small drug firm, the Massengill Company of Tennessee, following an intensive advertising campaign directed largely at physicians, put on sale the "Elixir of Sulfanilamide — Massengill." This was a raspberry-flavoured solution of sulfanilamide in the industrial liquid solvent, diethylene glycol. The composition of the "Elixir" was not stated on the label. In September and October of that year, 203 gallons were distributed in several southern states of the United States. During these months, physicians began observing small numbers of patients with uremia caused by unexplained shutdown of the kidneys. Those patients who were questioned admitted they were under treatment with Elixir of Sulfanilamide for a variety of infections. Autopsies done showed severe toxic damage to the kidneys. In many areas, the local health authorities and medical societies were notified; they in turn got in touch with the Federal Food and Drug Administration and the American Medical Association. These two organizations acted in co-operation quickly and effectively to terminate one of the largest mass poisonings ever to occur.

The existing law did not permit the authorities to discontinue the sale or shipment of drugs unless there was evidence of fraud, or unless the product failed to contain the substances itemized on the label. The FDA traced and seized all shipments and warned all involved of the hazard, employing the legal technicality that the product was not a true "elixir" — that is, the solvent was not alcohol, after the fashion of most elixirs. They could not charge at that time that the compound was dangerous or illegal because of a lack of proper prior testing. The American Medical Association released national warnings through radio and the press, urging physicians to report by wire collect any suspicious cases. The chemists and pharmacologists of the American Medical Association's Council on Pharmacy and Chemistry worked under pressure to analyze the drug and to determine on animals the toxicity of its components. They were able to prove that the solvent was diethylene glycol and that in small doses it produced severe damage to the kidney and death in rats, rabbits, and dogs. (Children had died after drinking less than an ounce.) The investigation disclosed that the "Elixir" had been tested by the Massengill Company for appearance, flavour, and fragrance, but not for safety.

Altogether, 358 persons were poisoned; 251 of these recovered; 107 died, many of them children. The chemist involved committed suicide. In a series of editorials, the *Journal of the American Medical Association* complained bitterly about the state of affairs which permitted drugs to be put on the market without being tested for toxicity. A lesson had been learned; the public outrage over this catastrophe was such that the proposed Food, Drug and Cosmetic Act of 1938, heretofore failing in Congress for lack of support, passed easily. This law required toxicity testing by the drug companies and gave the FDA the power it needed for seizure of products suspected of being hazardous to health. Not until twenty-four years later did the United States Government acquire the power to require evidence of effectivenss of drugs before they can be placed on the market.

Contaminated Yellow Fever Vaccine

The largest immunization catastrophe of all in terms of numbers of persons involved — 28,000 cases of hepatitis — is related to the use of yellow fever vaccine. In contrast with the Lübeck disaster caused by the administration of BCG for the prevention of tuberculosis, there was no mix-up or carelessness; in fact, every precaution then known was taken.

Epidemic yellow fever is one of the most dramatic and devastating of all the tropical diseases. Often referred to as a disease of the New World, it made its appearance in the 15th century following the early explorations and the opening of communications between Europe, America, and West Africa. In the 17th century, epidemics occurred in Spain, France, England, Italy, the entire Caribbean area, presumably resulting from the Aëdes aegyptii mosquito larvae in the water casks of the sailing ships. The legends of both the *Flying Dutchman* and the *Rime of the Ancient Mariner* are of ships stricken by yellow fever. As recently as 1905 serious outbreaks occurred in the southern United States, with 5,000 reported cases and 1,000 deaths.

In its epidemic form, yellow fever in some respects resembled the plagues described in Europe in the Middle Ages. People by the hundreds were suddenly stricken with fever; the attacks varied from mild to severe. Vomiting of blood was typical. Jaundice was the characteristic finding; hence the name "yellow fever," or "yellow jack." Patients either died or recovered in a matter of days. Thousands of deaths occurred in many outbreaks.

Carlos Finlay, a Cuban physician, recognized in 1881 that the mosquito propagated yellow fever. However, not until the turn of the century was this observation proven by the American Major Walter Reed and his commission, who used volunteer soldiers for the tests. This led to control of the disease by eliminating the mosquitoes, and by protecting the patiens from their bites. The measures taken indeed eliminated yellow fever and also greatly reduced the occurrence of malaria in Havana and Panama.

But sanitation alone could not eliminate the disease from large geographical areas. Yellow fever continued to smoulder in Central America, South America, and Africa. It lurked in the jungles, occasionally invading the towns and cities as an epidemic. In 1902 Walter Reed and James Carrol showed that the micro-organism was filterable and ultramicroscopic — the first proof that a filterable virus can cause a human disease. This discovery led to intensive research and extensive testing, involving thousands of animals, and subsequently the use of human volunteers, for an effective, safe vaccine. The attenuated vaccine became available for large-scale human application in 1938, one year before the beginning of the Second World War. More than 59,000 people were vaccinated in Brazil in 1939.

In the spring of 1942 cases of jaundice began appearing at army camps throughout the western United States. Reluctantly, the Army admitted the existence of a problem as the numbers rapidly increased. It became obvious that this was an epidemic of major proportions. The Surgeon General of the Army ordered full investigation and appointed an able team of experts to work on the problem. At first the nature of the disease was not apparent. There was nothing to distinguish it from the so-called catarrhal jaundice (more correctly designated infectious hepatitis) seen as scattered cases or small epidemics in the civilian population, except that this outbreak was more extensive and more sudden than anything experienced before. Most of the soldiers were only mildly ill. Laboratory tests excluded the common known micro-organisms which produce jaundice. A second possibility was that of exposure by military personnel to a toxic agent, such as an unsuspected poison. The third hypothesis, which seemed "fantastic" to most of the experts, was that of contamination of the human serum in yellow fever vaccine. There were previous experiences in England and Brazil with this vaccine; there the injection of certain lots had been followed by jaundice after a period of two to seven months.

A careful search for a toxic substance in the food, clothing, equipment, and medication used by the soldiers failed to disclose any possible common cause.

The epidemiologists on the team found no unusual amount of jaundice in any of the civilian communities adjacent to the involved army camps. There was no evidence of transmission by insects, food, or water supplies. The army camps were widely scattered over the western United States and Hawaii, with no apparent pattern of location or contact with previous cases. Nurses and doctors caring for patients did not acquire the disease. It did not spread.

Exploration of the third major possibility provided the answer as to the source of the problem. Nearly all the cases followed inoculation from only 9 of 177 lots of vaccine administered to nearly three million men, two to three months previously. Typhoid, small pox, and tetanus vaccines were eliminated as possible factors because of a wide variation in the time interval between vaccination and onset of jaundice.

The next effort of the investigating team was to establish how the harmful lots of vaccine produced the jaundice. Just as with tuberculosis, it had been found that only a greatly attenuated non-virulent living virus would act as an effective vaccine, and for that reason it could not be heat sterilized. In addition, it was thought necessary to add "normal" human serum obtained from "healthy" volunteers to preserve the attenuated yellow fever virus. This was also used because fewer reactions resulted from its application. Subsequently, it has been learned that an apparently normal, healthy person may harbour the living virus of serum hepatitis for long periods and can transmit it by injection of serum or blood to other human beings, but not to commonly used animals. Confirming evidence resulted from a painstaking investigation of the donors of the serum. The investigating team established that the human serum in the few lots of vaccine which seemed to have caused the jaundice were obtained for the most part from volunteers who had recovered from infectious hepatitis, and could therefore be carriers of the virus. It was soon found technically possible to produce a safe, effective serum-free yellow fever vaccine without using human serum. Hepatitis has not followed vaccination of tens of millions of persons since the human serum was omitted.

The *Journal of the American Medical Association* commented in an editorial in August 1942; "There is every reason to believe that vaccination against yellow fever is warranted and that the occurrence of 62 deaths and some 28,000 cases of jaundice is far less serious than would be an epidemic of virulent yellow fever among soldiers sent to the tropical areas in which our army is now engaging the enemy." Nevertheless, one wonders why it had been thought essential to immunize three million troops in a period of

15 months with a vaccine, certain lots of which could cause jaundice. The War Department certainly knew that a majority of the soldiers were not going to be sent to areas where they would be exposed to yellow fever.

Cutter Incident — Polio Vaccine

The third tragedy related to the administration of a useful vaccine may have occurred because of undue haste to use on a large scale a relatively new killed-virus vaccine.

Controlled field trials employing the newly developed Salk vaccine against paralytic polio were made on a large scale in 1954. Dr. Jonas Salk vaccinated 7,507 children with his vaccine with no harmful effect. Then more than 400,000 children were given commercially produced vaccine. The results indicated that the product was safe and effective. On April 2, 1955, polio vaccine was licensed for sale in the United States by the Secretary of Health, Education, and Welfare, upon the recommendation of the Surgeon General. After careful inspection of the plants, six well-known, established, reputable firms were permitted to make and sell the killed vaccine.

Some virologists and clinicians felt that this release was hasty and premature. During the last week of April 1955 a few cases of paralytic polio were reported in children vaccinated with material produced by one of the six firms, the Cutter Laboratories. A total of four million doses had been administered at this time.

Immediate steps were taken by the Surgeon General. All supplies of Cutter vaccine were withdrawn and all vaccinations halted until further information could be obtained on the quality and safety of all lots manufactured by the six firms. Later, after careful investigation, it was concluded that the paralysis of fifty-one vaccinated children and seventy-four family contact cases, was clearly related to use of the Cutter vaccine. There were ten deaths. The timing, the incidence, the geographic localization, the occurrence of paralysis in the inoculated arms, and the presence of live virus in some samples all indicated that the problem was limited to two of the eight batches of the material from the Cutter laboratory.

An exact answer to the nature of the error is lacking. The

systematic survey of each of the six plants involved revealed that the processes of inactivation of the viruses had been inconsistent in the hands of most of the manufacturers. The Surgeon General summarized this data as showing ". . . departures from the theoretical data, as well as a lack of discrimination in the previous testing practices." Salk and hs collaborator, Gori, feel that the original minimal requirements employed during the field trials had not been adhered to in detail in the manufacture of this complex biological material.

Lawsuits against Cutter were brought by many families whose children were involved. The laboratories were held legally responsible, though not negligent, and were required to pay a total of three million dollars.

As a result of this "incident," the minimum standards were revised; each of the six plants was inspected, with the production processes studied and the available supplies re-examined. Vaccination programs were resumed in the fall of the year under careful epidemiologic surveillance, and with tighter standards. Between the fall of 1955 and the end of 1961 over 400 million doses were administered, without evidence of production of polio by the inoculation. The 1958 World Health Organization report states; "Probably no new public health measure has ever been applied so rapidly on a mass scale after the laboratory research which led to its development." The overall result has been the disappearance of patients with the paralytic form of this disease in wards of children's hospitals throughout the world, to the gratification of all parents and doctors. In retrospect, it seems probable that more lives were saved than lost by the early use of the vaccine.

Since then, the Salk inactivated killed vaccine has been replaced by the effective live attenuated Sabin vaccine, which is given by mouth rather than by injection, and in contrast to the Salk vaccine, eliminates intestinal infection with polio virus and has a longer protective effect.

Coated Potassium Chloride Tablets

One of the most unusual of the laboratory mistakes was the one that resulted from the combination of two drugs and a coating.

In 1963 and 1964, patients began appearing in Minneapolis and in Stockholm with recurrent abdominal pain commencing one to three hours after a meal; often there was associated vomiting and weight loss. Frequently there was associated diarrhea and abdominal distention. The pain lasted minutes or hours, with intervals during which the patients were entirely without symptoms. A few patients had an acute illness and were admitted to hospial with severe abdominal pain and signs of peritonitis. The chronic recurrent cases usually became worse over a period of weeks or months and showed signs of intestinal obstruction with severe pains, vomiting, and abdominal distention. At first, in both the acute and chronic cases, the correct diagnosis was not suspected before the exploratory surgery was undertaken. Intestinal obstruction or perforation only were diagnosed.

At surgery, ulcers causing either secondary scarring and obstruction or perforation were found in the jejunum and ileum of the small intestine, well beyond the first portion, the duodenum, which connects with the stomach. While peptic ulcers in the duodenum are one of the most common of intestinal diseases, ulcers situated in the mid-portion of the small intestine are among the rarest. Surgical removal of the obstructed or perforated segment cured the condition and allowed careful examination of the ulcers, which were sharply limited areas five to ten millimeters across. There was no evidence of malignancy or infection. Because of the known rarity of a simple ulcer of this type, an epidemic was suspected. In Minneapolis and St. Paul, the records from twenty-five major hospitals were reviewed. No cases had been operated in 1960. Thereafter, there had been a rapid increase to twenty-seven in 1964. A similar review was made of the hospitals in the Stockholm area, where no cases were found between 1954 and 1957; then an increase in number was recorded, until the maximum of fifteen patients had surgery to relieve obstruction in 1964.

Nearly all of the patients were over fifty years of age (the mean age was sixty-two), with heart disease or high blood pressure. Most of the patients gave a history of receiving daily medication of two types — a thiazide and potassium chloride. In Minneapolis the physicians also noted that the potassium chloride had been in the form of tablets with a coating which did not dissolve until the tablet passed the stomach into the small intestine. The thiazide drugs were synthesized in 1957, and became available for use as valuable, effective agents for reducing high blood pressure, and for increasing the output of urine (diuretics), particularly for the relief of edematous accumulation of excess water in the body — a condition occurring in chronic heart failure. In 1960 this group of drugs was also found to be effective in the treatment of high blood pressure. Because of their effectiveness and the low toxicity of the tablets taken daily for months or years, they rapidly became widely used around the world. However, there was often the problem that along with flushing out the excess water, too much potassium was lost from the body, causing serious muscular weakness. This loss could be corrected by the addition of extra potassium by modifying the diet to include large amounts of fruit or potassium-containing salt substitutes. But it was simpler to give potassium chloride as medication whenever the thiazide therapy was intensive and continuous. Since both the liquid form of potassium chloride and uncoated tablets have an unpleasant taste and irritate the somach, coated tablets were produced in which the coating did not dissolve until the tablet reached the alkaline fluid of the small intestine. (This also avoided irritation of the stomach.)

At first it was suspected that the combination of a thiazide and the potassium chloride tablet produced the ulcers, but a series of studies on rabbits, dogs, and monkeys, undertaken in various countries in 1965 and 1966, quickly demonstrated that thiazide tablets alone, given by mouth, produced no ulcerations or inflammation of the stomach or intestines. Potassium chloride alone or in combination with thiazide gave rise to ulcers readily. The thiazide did not enhance the effect of the potassium chloride, but when the latter was administered, without the coating on the tablet, or as a highly concentrated solution, ulcers sometimes developed in the stomach; with the coating, the ulcers were localized in the small intestine. One group of investigators employed anchored with sutures coated tablets containing 1) a placebo, 2) thiazide, or 3) potassium chloride tablets and anchored them with sutures in the small intestines of dogs. At autopsy one to two weeks later, there were no remarkable changes at the sites where the placebos and thiazides had been placed. In segments containing the coated potassium chloride, the findings ranged from normal to ulceration, and even perforation, or gangrene. The microscopic findings indicated that the concentrated potassium chloride had caused occlusion of blood vessels and localized death of tissue. No animal studies had been submitted to the FDA prior to the release of the tablet, since it was assumed that previous experience with the separate ingredients made them unnecessary.

After the early reports from Minneapolis and Stockholm, many more cases from other geographic areas were reported in the next two years.

A large-scale survey of 440 hospitals disclosed 275 cases, with 15 deaths, in which the ulcers observed at surgery were definitely associated with use of the enteric-coated tablets. There were encouraging and unusual features in relation to his survey. The initial reports implicating thiazides and potassium chloride from Stockholm and Minneapolis had appeared in the fall of 1964. In November, representatives from the FDA and the two large drug firms involved — CIBA Pharmaceutical Company and Merck, Sharpe and Dohme — met to plan action to determine the prevalence of the obstructing ulcers in the small intestine, the deographic distribution of the cases, and the relationship of the ulcers to thiazides and poassium chloride. Within a month, the survey was completed and experiments on dogs and monkeys had confirmed that the enteric-coated tablets of potassium chloride were responsible for most of the ulcers. Warnings were issued at that time to take the tablets with meals and to discontinue them if there were abdominal pain. (It was apparent that the ulcers had occurred only rarely in proportion to the large numbers of people taking the drug.) Soon, however, tablets which slowly released the potassium chloride were substituted, and the epidemic ceased.

As the *Journal of the American Medical Association* pointed out at the time, the survey and the confirmatory tests done on animals represented an unusual example of effective co-operation of the medical profession, the pharmaceutical industry, and the Federal Government to control an epidemic. The surprising fact, in retrospect, is that the FDA did not at once compel the withdrawal from sale of this non-essential toxic preparation. Even in 1974 this product continued to be sold in the United States.

Hexachlorophene

The most recent of the laboratory mistakes and accidents is the tragedy occurring after the use of baby talcum powder containing hexachlorophene. This effective, non-irritating skin antiseptic has been used in most countries since its introducion thirty-three years ago. For several years it has been an ingredient of many creams, ointments, powders, cosmetics, antiperspirants, mouth washes, feminine deodorant sprays, toothpastes, and soaps. Its important use as Phisohex has been as a pre-operative skin preparation in surgery and in newborn nurseries, where it is effective in preventing epidemics of staphylococcal infections.

Ever since it was synthesized, it has been known to be toxic and potentially fatal if taken by mouth. In 1968 toxicity and deaths were reported from the use of hexachlorophene preparations on a few patients who had lost large areas of skin because of burns. Subsequently, researchers found that prolonged application to the skin on rats and monkeys could lead to central nervous system damage. Because of this finding, in December 1971 the FDA and the Committee on Fetus and Newborn of the American Academy of Pediatrics warned against its routine use in nurseries.

In the United States, many hospitals stopped total body bathing of newborns with hexachlorophene as a result of the warning by the FDA and the Academy of Pediatrics. Within three months there had been twenty-four outbreaks of staphylococcal infection related to discontinuance of the preparation. (There was no increase of such infections in fifty-eight other hospitals where such bathing had been continued.)

During the spring of 1972, 120 babies became seriously ill in various provinces of France, and 40 of them died. All had had a rash, which was followed by loss of appetite, irritability, drowsiness, twitching, and often convulsions. When death occurred, it arrived a few days after the onset of the illness. The only common factor which could be implicated was the use of "Talc Mohange," a baby talcum powder. In August 1972 the French Minister of Health announced that by accident a concentration of over 6 per cent hexachlorophene had been included in certain batches of the powder (3 per cent is the usual amount).

Lessons of caution have been learned. An essential drug known to be toxic in higher than usual doses should be handled with caution and respect, but should not be discontinued unless it can be suitably replaced — a delicate balance between risk and benefit.

At present, the usual practice is to use it on only full-term infants, and to rinse off the residue thoroughly with water. Premature babies are washed with it only if threatened by an epidemic of staphylococcal infection.

CHAPTER THREE

Side Effects of Drugs

It is now well recognized that all drugs have toxic or side effects, and that it is the ratio of benefit to risk that decides the value of the medication used. (The same principle holds for surgery and the use of x-ray and radioactive materials.) Even penicillin, one of the safest and most effective of drugs, has caused several hundred deaths in the United States. But in the case of penicillin, it is obvious that the benefit — often life saving — to millions clearly outweighs this risk. In the situations cited below, the ratio was reversed. Toxic side effects following usual treatment were clearly greater than the benefits, and the use of these drugs for the diseases discussed has been discontinued.

Four of the errors analyzed in this presentation produced ill effects in the offspring of the mothers treated during pregnancy. In three examples, teratogenic ("monster-causing") effects of the drugs — synthetic progestins, thalidomide, and Vitamin D (*cf* Chapter IV, *Overdose*) — resulted in congenital malformations. In the fourth, the use of stilbestrol produced cancer of the vagina in the daughters, when the latter reached their teens.

Teething Powders and Laxatives — Pink Disease

Of all the diseases resulting from treatment, acrodynia (meaning pain in the extremities) required the most time for the recognition of its true nature.

Acrodynia, or pink disease, had been observed in 1890 and well described in 1903, but not until almost half a century later, in 1948, did Warkany and Hubbard publish their classic paper indicating that it was a form of chronic mercury poisoning.

All doctors caring for children during this period were aware of the easily distinguishable and highly characteristic condition. The typical patient was a sweating, fretful, miserable, restless infant or young child, with pink hands and feet, suffering from itching, burning, severe pain of the extremities, and marked sensitivity to light. Inflammation of the mouth, with red swollen gums and excessive production of saliva, were common; occasionally there was a loss of hair, teeth, nails, and even fingers and toes. Most patients recovered after months of illness; about one in twenty died. Between 1939 and 1948 a total of 585 children died from this disease in Wales and England alone, and thousands of cases were believed to have occurred in the first half of the century, there and elsewhere.

Geographically, there was an unusual pattern, in that the disease appeared in certain areas, varying widely in frequency from one year to another. It was particularly common in parts of Australia, northwestern United States, most of England, and much of continental Europe, with no especial significance regarding distribution of cases.

Many possibilities were considered in the search for a cause, including vitamin deficiencies, viral encephalitis, and toxic reactions (arsenic was most often suspected). In 1947 Fanconi and his coworkers in Switzerland suggested that mercury might be the cause. The following year, Warkany and Hubbard demonstrated the presence of excess mercury in urine of children with acrodynia, and proceeded to piece together the evidence that the disease is due to a low tolerance to mercurial medications, existing in a minority of children. Warkany, in a fine historical account entitled "Acrodynia — a Post Mortem," tells the story. He and others had suspected arsenic, which causes similar symptoms and which sometimes contaminates wine and beer; it is also used in many industrial applications. In addition, he had a laboratory available in which a variety of metal determinations could be performed on blood and urine samples. The chemist, Mr. Hubbard, had devised a test for the determination of mercury in the urine in 1940. After learning in several cases that there was no excess arsenic, Warkany requested "qualitative metal determinations," hoping that a metal other than arsenic might be discovered. Lead, aluminum, copper, silver, thallium, cobalt, antimony, manganese, and mercury were sought. The high level of mercury found in the urine was also present in 120 of the 189 urine samples obtained over the next four years, from children with acrodynia. Only two of eighty-seven control samples showed large amounts of mercury. A history of exposure to mercury was obtained in the few cases in which the urine samples were free of excess mercury. However, there was a problem. The samples from patients with acrodynia were sent from all over the United States; the samples from the controls were gathered from Cincinnati, where both the disease and the use of mercurial medications were rare.

In London in 1951 significant amounts of mercury were recovered from eleven patients and fifteen out of sixteen control urines. This had the unfortunate effect of postponing the withdrawal in England of the mercury-containing teething powders and other medications, from widespread use for children.

Once mercury was suspected, another look was taken at the epidemiological facts. In the British Commonwealth, most of the patients were infants around nine months of age; the disease seldom occurred in those over two years of age. In Europe, most children were around three years, and many cases occurred up to the age of nine. This difference could be explained by the fact that in British countries, mercury in the form of calomel (mercurous chloride) in teething powders was used for infants; in Europe, calomel was extensively used as a laxative and as a worming medicine for young children. In both forms, its use was widespread. The additional bit of circumstantial evidence was the abrupt decline of the numbers of cases, when restrictive laws were passed in Australia in 1953. In 1959 in Adelaide, where the disease had formerly been common, only one case occurred. Similarly, in Switzerland and the United States, the incidence of the disease sharply dropped when the use of calomel decreased. (Almst thirty years elapsed before the United States Food and Drug Administration could influence manufacturers to completely remove mercury from the teething powders.)

In England, where no organized effort was made to eliminate the use of calomel in children's preparations, the disease lingered on, gradually disappearing only as the drug houses discontinued the use of calomel, and as the product disappeared from the shelves of the grocers and chemists. Occasional cases still occurred in 1966.

The delayed recognition of the association of mercury with acrodynia is understandable on the basis of the fact that when children are exposed, only a minority develop the disease (Warkany estimated 1 in 500), and then, only after a lag of weeks to months. In addition, in acrodynia, poisoning occurred from various medications — mercury in the form of ointments, teething powders, worm medicines, laxatives, diaper rinses. This often made it difficult or impossible to obtain a history of exposure to mercury. Finally, the typical findings of mercurial acrodynia were never produced in animals.

On the other hand, as Warkany points out, a good knowledge of medical history should have led clinicians to suspect the association long before. The use of mercury in medicine has a long and fascinating history dating back a thousand years, to its use by Arabian physicians in the form of ointments for chronic skin diseases, leprosy, and typhus. These physicians described the profuse sweating resulting from mercury poisoning. Later, when epidemics of syphilis appeared in Europe shortly after the voyages of Columbus, mercury was found to be the only agent in any way effective against the disease, remaining so until the 1800s. Mercurial treatments were pushed to the point at which patients developed not only sweating, but also excessive production of saliva, soreness of the mouth, swollen gums, and loss of teeth — all characterstic signs of acrodynia in infants and young children. It is probable that had this knowledge of past experience been applied, recognition of the association of mercury and acrodynia might have appeared years earlier.

Silver Antiseptics — Blue-Grey Skin

Silver and silver compounds have been used as medicines since ancient times. In the 18th century, the condition of argyria (from the Greek *argyro,* "silver"), a slate blue discolouration of the skin, was described in patients receiving chronic treatment with silver preparations. More reports followed, and the condition became widely recognized. But in the second half of the 19th century, because of less faith in the value of these medications and increased fear of the disease on the part of physicians, argyria became rare.

In 1889 silver preparations were shown to have strong antiseptic action when applied locally. The simple salts, such as silver nitrate, were astringent and irritating, but it became possible to make organic preparations combining the metal with colloid compounds employing proteins, producing effective local antiseptics which slowly liberated silver ions and were non-irritating when applied to mucous membranes. These included the trade preparations Argyn, Silvol, Neo-Silvol, Solargentum, and Argyrol, all of which came to have a widespread use both by prescription and as home remedies bought over the counter. They were sprayed, swabbed, and used as an irrigating agent on the membranes of the throat, the sinuses, the bladder, the vagina and the colon. Often their use was the result of efforts to rid the body of focal infection; chronic use for periods of years was commonplace. Some advertisers falsely claimed that their products would not cause argyria.

Between 1900 and 1940, over 100 cases of argyria were reported from European countries and North America; many more undoubtedly occurred. All physicians were said to have seen one or more patients with the disease, but most went unrecorded. Deposits of silver occurred in almost all organs of the body as well as the skin, but, surprisingly, seemed to do no harm to health. The discolouration was bluish in the parts of the body exposed to light, while the rest of the skin appeared a slate grey. The disagreeably unhealthy appearance, remaining permanently, caused serious harm to psyche and personality. Some patients refused to go out of doors in daylight or to mingle with others.

In retrospect there seem to have been no beneficial effects from the *chronic* treatments, except that the inventor of Argyrol, who became a millionaire, endowed one of the world's finest museums of impressionist art.

A Depilatory – Poisoning and Death

In the present treatment of cancer, many toxic drugs with known serious side effects are used deliberately because it is felt that the hazards of such treatment are justfied. However, in the use of thallium and, later, dinitrophenol, known poisons were employed for relatively minor conditions — ringworm of the scalp, undesired hair on face or body, and for obesity — all of which could be effectively treated by other methods.

Thallium, discovered in 1861, is one of the most toxic of metals, the salts of which are used to kill rats and ants. It is, therefore, one of the most dangerous drugs. At the turn of the century, it was noted that one of its highly characteristic toxic effects is alopecia, or loss of hair. To remove hair, dermatologists began making trials of ointments to be applied locally, and medications to be given by mouth in doses sufficiently low, so they hoped, to avoid the other unpleasant toxic effects which included nausea, vomiting, cramps, weakness, staggering, burning and tingling of hands and feet, paralysis, coma, and occasionally, death. But not until the 1920s did thallium as the acetate salt come into common use for treatment of ringworm of the scalp in children. It was given by mouth in a single dose; the loss of the infected hairs, occurring in two to three weeks, cured the disease. The treatment was simple and popular, particularly in orphan homes and institutions for the mentally retarded, where ringworm was an irksome, though not serious, problem. Many dermatologists used the treatment enthusiastically, though warning against its indiscriminate use.

In 1931 thallium acetate was introduced as a depilatory cream for cosmetic use, under the trade name Koremulu.

During the late 1920s and early 1930s, cases of poisoning and deaths were reported from many countries, both from the oral medication and the cream. By 1934, Munch was able to collect from the literature and from colleagues, records of 692 cases of poisoning and 31 deaths from the medicinal use of thallium. It was thought that there were many more not reported. Poisoning seemed to have occurred in about 5 per cent of the children who had been properly treated. The promoters of Koremulu underwent bankruptcy because of many lawsuits, and the preparation was taken off the market. Thereafter, thallium poisoning from medicinal use gradually became rare; most cases were due to children eating it in the form of rat poison.

The few animal experiments made had shown that the drug was harmful, but no controlled clinical trials were reported.

A Headache Powder and Pain Reliever —
Disease of the White Blood Cells

One of the early epidemics involving a synthetic drug did not appear for a quarter of a century after its introduction.

Beginning in 1922 case reports began appearing of what seemed to be a new disease, manifested by fever, extreme soreness and inflammation of the mouth and throat with associated infection and ulcerations, and a characteristic severe depression in the numbers of circulating white blood cells. Because of these blood changes, the disease was termed agranulocytosis (absence of granular cells). Most patients died from it, and those who did were found at autopsy to have evidence of marked toxic effects on the bone marrow, which produces the white blood cells. While the few initial cases were reported from Germany, soon reports appeared from other countries — England, Denmark, Belgium, Switzerland, and the United States. However, there was considerable variation in the incidence of the disease from country to country. Because of the severe inflammation of the mouth and throat, the associated fever and the frequent findings of bacteria in the blood, agranulocytosis was for almost a decade assumed to be probably the result of primary overwhelming bacterial infection, though the possibilities of a reaction to a toxic agent or an atypical form of leukemia were often mentioned.

By 1931 about 200 cases had been reported. That year an American pathologist, Robert Kracke, called attention to a number of pertinent facts: the disease occurred only in Europe and the United States; the incidence was largest among middle-aged white women living under good economic conditions; many of the patients were physicians, nurses, technicians, or wives of doctors; most patients had a history of care or treatment with various drugs. Kracke reasoned that except for laxatives, the most common drugs in use at that time in that part of the world were those synthetics derived from coal tars with chemical molecules containing benzene rings. He had already demonstrated experimentally that agranulocytosis could be produced in rabbits by injecting benzene in olive oil under the skin. He tried unsuccessfully to produce the disease in animals by giving by mouth and by injection a variety of drugs containing rings of the benzene molecule — among them, amidopyrine.

Two years later, two Americans, Madison and Squier, produced conclusive evidence that the pain- and headache-relieving drug, amidopyrine, containing a benzene ring, could produce agranulocytosis. They reported fourteen patients in whom the onset of the disease was directly preceded by the use of amidopyrine alone, or in combination with a barbiturate. They concluded that the drug alone was capable of producing the disease in certain sensitive individuals allergic to the drug. Their conclusions were supported by the fact that the administration of single ordinary doses to two patients who had recovered from the disease precipitated a temporary marked depression of the numbers of white cells in the blood, which did not occur after giving the barbiturate. Their observations were confirmed by others. However, it soon became known that other drugs — the gold compounds used in tuberculosis, dinitrophenol employed to prevent obesity, salvarsan for syphilis, and later, sulfanilamide — could also produce agranulocytosis, though less often. Kracke's theory about the benzene ring may have been wrong, but he was right about the drug toxicity as a cause of the disease.

Amidopyrine was synthesized in 1893, introduced in Europe in 1897, and appeared on the American market around 1909. Like aspirin and phenacetin, amidopyrine is an effective pain reliever, relieving aches and reducing the temperature in fever. Also like the other two drugs, it soon became tremendously popular and widely used, combined with barbiturates frequently, and incorporated into many proprietary remedies for headaches, muscular pains, colds, and rheumatic conditions. After 1931 the numbers of cases of agranulocytosis steadily increased. Between the years 1931 and 1934 the Department of Vital Statistics recorded 1,981 deaths from agranulocytosis in the United States. By far the most commonly associated drug (80 per cent) in all the reports at that time was amidopyrine. A Danish investigator was able to correlate the incidence of the disease with the sales of the drug in Denmark, and to show that the increase in cases paralled its increased use. In England in 1936 amidopyrine was allowed as a prescription drug; in the United States, it was removed from the lists of official drugs in 1938. Its sale dropped markedly, and, by 1940, reports of lethal cases attributable to its use became rare. But in spite of the fact that all medical texts warned against its use, a total of sixty-five cases of agranulocytosis associated with the use of the drug in the United States between 1957 and 1964 were reported. This may have been due to the fact that some mixtures issued under a proprietary name contained amidopyrine without the knowledge of the prescribing physician, since in Denmark, when amidopyrine had been taken completely out of use in the late 1930s, no cases were reported between 1951 and 1957.

A curious, unsettled problem remains. Several estimates showed that among Americans, English, and Danes who had consumed significant amounts of the drug, approximately 1 per cent developed agranulocytosis, whereas in Germany, the figure stood at only 0.1 per cent. In Spain, where amidopyrine is still readily available, it is said that no cases have been reported. The occasional British tourist on vacation in these countries does develop agranulocytosis after taking the drug. This type of idiosyncrasy may be due to genetic differences, for allergic tendencies are often inherited.

Gold in Tuberculosis — Disease of the White Blood Cells

Gold in the treatment of tuberculosis was a form of drug therapy greeted with enthusiasm and widely used when it first appeared in 1925, largely given up when two limited but carefully planned controlled studies demonstrated its lack of value and serious toxicity, but not entirely abandoned until fifteen years after its introduction, when it was replaced by truly effective treatment.

In 1882 Robert Koch, the great German bacteriologist, established without question that the tubercle bacillus was the one essential cause of tuberculosis — the major cause of death from disease in industrial countries at that time. This stimulated an intense search for methods of treatment. Among the many agents Koch tested were certain gold salts. He found that these would inhibit the growth of the bacteria in the test tube even in very high dilutions, although they did not cure experimentally infected animals. Subsequently, other investigators continued to try other gold compounds on animals, with variable effect, mostly discouraging.

However, Paul Ehrlich had devised his magic bullet — "606," salvarsan — for the treatment of relapsing fever, yaws, and syphilis. This ushered in the era of chemotherapy in 1909 with the concept that it was possible to deliberately synthesize substances toxic to infecting organisms and harmless to their hosts. It led to continued searching for other agents in other diseases and stimulated reconsideration of the gold compounds for the treatment of tuberculosis. A Danish professor of physiology at the Royal Veterinary and Agricultural College in Copenhagen, Holger Moellgaard, in 1925 published a monograph entitled *Chemotherapy of Tuberculosis,* and the age of gold treatment began. The drug, called sanocrysin, was sodium gold thiosulphate, a chemical isolated in the middle of the 19th century and used by Daguerre in developing the first photographs. Moellgaard believed it was a true magic bullet, in the sense that it had an affinity for the parasite, and that, when introduced into the blood stream, it permeated the tuberculosis foci and destroyed most or all of the offending tubercle bacilli. He claimed that the compound had been effective in saving the lives of goats, calves, and monkeys which were "gravely infected." The preliminary results on human beings obtained by his Danish clinical colleagues were equally encouraging. Early acute, progressive pulmonary disease was considered the form most likely to respond.

Within two years the drug was widely used around the world with varying results. There is such a wide fluctuation in the clinical course of human tuberculosis — many patients recover spontaneously, many have relapses over a period of years, many die after a long or short illness — that it is particularly difficult to evaluate the results of treatment. For the most part, the reports of good results were based on comparisons with previous results of other treatment in patients assumed to be similar, or on enthusiastic testimonials of outstanding results in individual cases. The Danish workers claimed that 52 per cent of patients were cured or improved. Within a few years, and after the initial acceptance, an increasing number of reports of toxic reactions began to appear, including severe skin eruptions, damage to kidney and liver, depression of the bone marrow function in the production of white cells (agranulocytosis), and occasional deaths. All these reactions seemed to be due to the drug rather than the disease, for the use of gold salts at that time in rheumatoid arthritis and syphilis produced the same untoward effects. A British Medical Research Council report published in 1926 analyzed the results of treating 140 patients in 14 hospitals throughout the United Kingdom. The findings were inconclusive, though several observers felt that sanocrysin was of definite value in certain cases. Three deaths in this series were ascribed to the drug. Two small but carefully controlled clinical trials were made; the first, reported in 1931 from Detroit, included twenty-four carefully selected and closely comparable patients. The group was divided at random into twelve controls and twelve patients treated with sanocrysin. All ancillary treatment was identical; the patients were cared for concurrently, and it was single-blind, in that the patients were unaware of any distinction in the treatment administered. The conclusions were that there was no evidence clinically or from the laboratory findings of a beneficial effect on pulmonary tuberculosis or its complications. On the contrary, compared with the controls, more of the sanocrysin-treated cases became worse. The drug produced harmful effects on nutrition and on gastrointestinal and kidney function. One treated patient died of severe liver disease, which on autopsy examination appeared to be due to the gold.

Two English physicians in 1935 reported similar results among patients sixteen to twenty-six years old treated over a five-year period. The two groups were larger, but though carefully carried out, the trial was by no means ideal. The physicians found that differences between the control and treated groups were statistically negligible. Their comment is still pertinent: "The examination of our statistical results has been a painful shock, for we were convinced whilst carrying out this costly method of treatment that in chrysotherapy [gold therapy] we had found a valuable aid; many of the cases seemed to do extremely well. But one tends to forget that many cases previously did extremely well even without gold. It is to us a sad reminder of the extreme fallibility of clinical judgment when exposed to the cruel light of a controlled statistical inquiry on a large number of cases."

In spite of these two studies and the increasing numbers of papers appearing in medical journals describing toxic effects, sanocrysin continued to be used in selected cases, particularly in Europe.

The discovery in 1944 by Selman Waksman of streptomycin, a product of a soil fungus systematically sought after, began the first truly effective chemotherapy for tuberculosis. Its low toxicity in experimental animals, together with the promising results in treating infected guinea pigs, was encouraging. Also, two years later the product kept alive some patients suffering from tuberculous meningitis, previously always fatal. It has been repeatedly pointed out that almost the only circumstance in which a controlled trial is unnecessary in studying the treatment of any disease is one in which the disease, under existing treatment, uniformly results in death. In 1947 a series of carefully controlled large-scale, well-planned and co-ordinated clinical trials was carried out over a period of ten years, under the auspices of the British Medical Research Council. At the same time, similar studies were made by the United States Public Health Service and the Veterans Administration in the United States. Many lessons had been learned from the failures of the past. Combinations of treatment had to be compared when the new drugs isoniazid and PAS (para-amino salicyclic acid) became available, and it was necessary to observe patients for years to evaluate the results.

While a double-blind study was often not possible (one treatment had to be injected; another taken by mouth), concurrent treatment and random allocation of patients with disease of similar severity and type were made. The radiologists assessing x-ray changes in pulmonary tuberculosis were kept unaware of the treatment. Because of the wide variability in the course of the disease, large numbers of patients were involved. By 1957 highly effective treatment using a combination of streptomycin, isoniazed and PAS had been established on a firm basis. (Resistance to a single remedy or drug may develop.) Where treatment has been available, tuberculosis has been conquered, and this conquest has been one of the finest and most important accomplishments in the entire history of medicine.

A Reducing Pill — Cataract

An outbreak of eye cataracts began in the spring of 1935, chiefly in the United States but also in most European countries and Brazil.

It increased to a peak in the fall of that year, and gradually disappeared in 1937. Characteristically, the victims were healthy young women who were obese and who had been receiving dinitrophenol, taken for the rapid reduction of weight. A total of 177 cases were reported — the largest number of any toxic epidemic of cataracts until that time.

The ill effects of dinitrophenol, an explosive related to trinitrotluene (TNT), were well known, having been a problem among the French munitions workers during the First World War. Near the turn of the century investigators had shown the substance to accelerate the metabolism of animals, sometimes causing death with high fever. There was a wide variation in reactions of animals, even of the same species.

In 1931 a group of pharmacologists and clinicians at Stanford University began extensive studies and trials, first on animals and later on humans. Their efforts led them to the conclusion two years later that dinitrophenol in doses "not demonstrably harmful" markedly increased the metabolism of the body thereby causing weight loss. The experimenters recognized that the drug was dangerous and advocated further careful trials on patients. Later that year they urged its general use under supervision of physicians, calling it "relatively safe." The Stanford group treated 113 obese patients conntinuously up to four months without serious side effects, and with success. Many patients became slightly yellow because of the colour of the drug itself. They usually sweated profusely because of their increased metabolic rate.

An overwhelming popular response by physicians and patients ensued. A simple answer seemed available for all who were overweight and suffering from fatigue due to "low metabolism." It is probable that over a million persons took the drug, which could be bought under a variety of trade names without prescription from any one of twenty drug houses. Dinitrophenol was advertised to both physicians and the public as "absolutely safe when taken in accordance with directions."

Soon reports of serious toxic reactions in patients taking the drug began to appear in the medical journals. These reactions consisted chiefly of skin rashes, often with intense itching and depression of the bone marrow, involving principally the white blood cells (agranulocytosis). Nine deaths occurred. But not until 1935 were cataracts described. Their occurrence was surprising, since no cataracts had appeared in the laboratory animals given various and repeated doses of dinitrophenol. The number of patients with cataracts increased rapidly. Horner, in his narrative account, estimated that up to 1 per cent of those receiving the drug lost their vision. The interval between cessation of medication and the development of cataract was up to one year, and the damage was permanent, though operative treatment was successful in most cases. The circumstantial evidence was strong, and no other cause could be demonstrated.

Reaction set in. In 1935 the German Federal Bureau of Health warned against the use of dinitrophenol; Canada banned its sale. In the next year England restricted it to sale by prescription only. In the United States the response was slower. Not until October 1936 did the *Journal of the American Medical Association,* which had been uneasy about the drug since its introduction in 1933, take a strong stand and warn against its use in obesity. (Their council of pharmacy and chemistry never approved it.) In the United States, only individual states took legislative action. Many of them ruled that dinitrophenol could be sold by prescription only. California was unique in that in 1939 a law was passed making it a felony to sell or prescribe the drug for human consumption, within the state. Until 1938 the United States' Government could take no action except to bar it from the mails when the advertising was fraudulent. Then, empowered by the new legislation requiring manufacturers to prove the safety of any new drug, the F.D.A. forced it off the market.

Just as with thallium, dinitrophenol appears to be another example of the unjustified use on a large scale, and after inadequate clinical trials, of a drug known to be highly toxic, in treatment of a condition usually not serious, which could be treated by other means.

Synthetic Hormones — Masculinization of Daughters

The first of the three congenital malformations occurring as a result of the use of the drugs discussed in this presentation was the unusual effect on the fetus after the use of synthetic progesterone hormones during pregnancy.

In 1950 at Johns Hopkins University Hospital, Lawson Wilkins, a pediatric endocrinologist, and Howard Jones, a gynecologist, began noticing in the endocrine clinic a few female infants and young girls with masculinized external genitals and normal female internal genitalia (vagina, uterus, fallopian tubes, overies). In most instances the patients were recognized to be girls, but were brought in because the clitoris so resembled a penis that some form of hermaphroditism was suspected. There was often in addition fusion of the labia, obstructing the vaginal opening. (In a few instances, the children were reared as boys until adolescence, when breast development and other secondary sex characteristics made it evident that they were girls.) Wilkins and his group were able to demonstrate by chromosomal material from cells of the mucous membrane of the mouth that the patients were genetically female. The term "pseudo-hermaphroditism" was applied. They also proved by chemical analysis of the urine that there was no excess production nor excretion of male sex hormones in these patients. The surgical exposure through an incision in the abdomen in eight of the early cases revealed the presence of normal internal genitalia — uterus, fallopian tubes, and ovaries. Many of the patients required plastic surgical correction of the external abnormalities. A review of the medical literature revealed only twelve previously reported similar cases.

Other investigators confirmed in other species the fact that most of the synthetic progestins were masculinizing, and that all masculinizing hormones could produce these effects on the female offspring. In five of the twelve previously reported cases of pseudohermaphroditism, the mothers had received male sex hormones for various illnesses during their pregnancies. The probable cause was quickly apparent to Wilkins and Jones, once these facts were known. They questioned the mothers of their patients and learned that all but three of them had received hormonal treatment with progestins early in pregnancy, for threatened abortion. In view of all this evidence the investigators concluded that there was a probable causal association between the use of the progestins and the malformation and reported their findings at a national conference on hormones.

Progesterone is one of the two major female sex hormones secreted by the ovary. The word itself means "to favour pregnancy," and the function of the hormone is chiefly to prepare the lining of the uterus for the fertilized ovum and to maintain normal pregnancy. Hence it seemed logical to use progestins, the synthetic derivatives, for threatened spontaneous abortion, as it was assumed, without adequate evidence, that many of these women suffered from a deficiency of progesterone. The accepted practice of using the injectable progesterone from the natural sources for this purpose led to the widespread use of synthetic derivatives, the progestins, when they became available, in the late forties. The natural product could be given only by injection; the synthetic progestins could be administered by mouth.

After the publication of the initial findings of Wilkins and Jones and their co-workers in 1958, a host of reports followed, confirming the original findings. Nearly 600 female babies were born with varying degrees of masculinized genitalia.

Previous investigations, beginning in 1939 in animals, proved that some of the synthetic progestins having molecular structures similar to the potent male sex hormone testosterone have strong masculinizing effects on various animal species. Two French endocrinologists, Courcier and Jost, had already reported in 1942 that the administration of the first synthetic progestins to pregnant rabbits resulted in masculinization of the external genitalia in some of the female offspring. They warned about this occurrence as a possible hazard if this synthetic drug were given to women for threatened abortion, but their warning went unheeded.

Because the defects when severe were surgically correctible, at first Wilkins and Jones urged only caution in treating mothers with the progestins then employed, limiting the dose and restricting its use to cases in which hormonal deficiency was proven. Yet, even after both warnings, large pharmaceutical companies continued to advertise these drugs as safe during pregnancy.

Later, in 1950, two well-controlled studies were conducted in groups of women who habitually aborted and who had evidence of progesterone deficiency. There was no evidence of a beneficial effect of these drugs. Yet, because the toxic effects were uncommon in proportion to the number of women treated (less than 1 per cent), and because there was no other satisfactory treatment then, a few obstetricians were reluctant to give them up, even though current textbooks decried their use. There followed a sharp decline of cases reported concurrent with decreased use of all hormone medication during pregnancy.

While this epidemic was far less devastating than the phocomelia produced by the teratogenic drug, thalidomide, it also serves to illustrate the hazards of the use of drugs during pregnancy.

A Treatment for Boils — Encephalitis

The second of the episodes of mass poisonings due to gross neglect was that which resulted from the use of a highly toxic tin di-iodide compound in the treatment of infections.

Physicians in various areas of France in 1954 began seeing patients who had become acutely ill, with headache, vomiting, cramps, prostration, and often loss of vision —signs of toxic encephalitis. It was quickly recognized that the patients had been under treatment for staphylococcal infections — usually boils — and that the medication they all had been receiving was stalinon (di-ethyl tin di-iodide), which a pharmacist in a small town near Paris had recently put on the market. Before the drug was withdrawn the same year, 217 persons were poisoned, and 110 died.

The metal tin in itself is practically non-toxic; but in combination with the organic iodide as stalinon it was shown in the same year (1954) by English investigators to be highly toxic to animals. In addition, previous tests in 1931 had demonstrated it to be ineffective against boils and other staphylococcal infections. The French pharmacist himself, unaware of this information, had failed to test this product on animals, before marketing it.

A Cholesterol Reducing Agent —
Cataract, Loss of Hair, and Impotence

The only large-scale medical blunder which appears to have been made as a result of deliberate deception was that related to the use of triparanol, called by the proprietary name MER/29, produced by the William S. Merrell Company.

In April 1961 physicians at the Mayo Clinic observed six patients who developed loss of hair, and dry, scaling skin while under treatment with a new drug, triparanol. Nineteen patients were receiving treatment. The changes were so unusual that the clinicians suspected a causal relationship between the drug and the observed symptoms. Later that same year cases of unexplained cataract occurring in patients on the drug were reported to the Merrell Company, which issued a warning statement about this hazard but took no further action at that time. However, because of an increased number of reports of these and other reactions, including impotence, loss of hair, vomiting, and female breast development in male patients, the company, under pressure, withdrew the drug from the market early in 1962. Subsequently, reports of cataracts and other reactions rapidly increased in number — manifestations often delayed for up to a year after the drug was discontinued. It was estimated that about 1 per cent of the patients receiving the drug suffered toxic effects.

One of the most-needed drugs is an effective agent to prevent or treat arteriosclerosis — now the greatest single cause of premature death in industrial countries throughout the world. For many years it has been recognized that patients who died in middle age of heart attacks due to coronary arteriosclerosis usually had increased amounts of cholesterol in their blood; conversely, those with low levels rarely had heart attacks before old age. The higher the level, the greater the risk. In addition, much experimental evidence indicated a strong causal relationship. It was shown that a strict diet very low in animal fats would reduce the level; but the diet was so unpleasant that most people would not adhere to it. There ensued a vigorous search for an effective drug of low toxicity which would produce the same result. The unproven assumption was that lowering the cholesterol would prevent heart attacks, thus prolonging life. Among the many drugs considered, one showing great promise was a newly developed synthetic organic compound, triparanol, produced by ingenious chemical manipulation of the molecular structure. It reduced the concentration of cholesterol in the blood, liver, and other tissues of experimental animals by inhibiting its synthesis in the body. This drug was developed and tested in the laboratories of the William S. Merrell pharmaceutical company in Cincinnati, Ohio, in 1958. Tests for acute, subacute and chronic toxicity were made on rats, dogs, and monkeys. Triparanol in effective doses was said to not interfere with growth. Careful autopsy findings were reported as not revealing serious ill effects, and the margin of safety was said to be "comfortable." Function studies on living monkeys indicated that the drug did not interfere with liver function nor the bone marrow activity in the production of red cells and white cells.

Most preliminary clinical trials on small numbers of patients at several centres indicated that patients with arteriosclerosis of the coronary arteries and the arteries in the legs showed a reduction in the blood cholesterol levels and clinical improvement, after receiving one or two of the mouse-grey capsules daily for a period of months. Anginal pains were frequently relieved; patients experienced less shortness of breath and enjoyed improved exercise tolerance and well-being. However, little objective evidence of improvement was noticed in the electrocardiograms, and some studies failed to demonstrate even symptomatic improvement. Only one controlled clinical trial appears to have been done. This indicated that MER/29 had failed to cause improvement in a small number of patients. All of this information was presented and discussed at a symposium on the subject of MER/29, sponsored by the Merrell Company, at Princeton, New Jersey, in December 1959. The participants included some of the most distinguished scientists and clinicians in the United States. The papers presented were promptly published in the new but well-regarded journal *Progress in Cardiovascular Disease* early in 1950. The editor made it clear that the publication did not imply approval or disapproval of the new drug; the wide circulation of the journal did provide the medication with great publicity, most of it favourable.

Shortly thereafter, the drug was released by the FDA for general prescription use, with only a few objections. But those few included some from scientists at the National Heart Institute, a pharmacologist at the FDA itself, and the *Medical Letter,* which provides expert objective evaluation of drugs. Hundreds of thousands of patients received it, many of them with no apparent disease other than elevation of the blood cholesterol. Triparanol was given in the hope of preventing coronary heart disease and other effects of arteriosclerosis, in spite of the fact that there was no factual evidence to indicate that the drug would accomplish this. It has been estimated that a thousand individuals developed cataract as a result of this treatment. Additional further investigation revealed that it was of doubtful value in preventing or reducing arteriosclerosis. In blocking synthesis of cholesterol in the liver, an accumulation of the chemical desmosterol resulted. This concerned investigators, because they felt it to be as injurious as cholesterol, or more so. More importantly, triparanol was never evaluated by the employment of a planned, large-scale, controlled clinical trial, to determine its effectiveness and toxicity. There appears little question that it was made available prematurely for general use by well-intentioned physicians.

Worst of all was the fact that a cover-up existed. According to Walter Modell, editor of the journal *Clinical Pharmacology and Therapeutics,* "Critical laboratory data on triparanol were criminally suppressed. Pharmacological tests in the laboratories of the manufacturer of triparanol had shown that in rats and dogs, cataract formation, loss of hair, and gonadal changes occurred. Thus the effects that were subsequently seen in man — cataracts, loss of hair, and impotence — were predicted by laboratory observations but suppressed." The firm was fined \$80,000 by the District Court in Washington, D.C., for withholding and falsifying test data.

Thalidomide — Deformed Children, Polyneuritis

The most spectacular and widely known of the drug disasters of this century was the world-wide calamity produced by the use of the sedative thalidomide. More than ten years have passed since the tragedy; hence it is possible to give a reasonably objective account. Briefly, the chronology is as follows:

1956 — Thalidomide sold under the trade name Contergan was marketed in Germany as a safe, effective non-toxic, sleep-producing sedative drug. Tests on animals (mice, rats, rabbits, dogs, and monkeys), all indicated that large amounts given as a single dose caused no ill effects. Uncontrolled clinical trials indicated it was safe and effective in producing sleep and tranquility in man.

1960-61 — Case reports appearing in the medical journals of polyneuritis with accounts of the tingling, itching, burning, and weakness of the legs and arms of patients given thalidomide daily over a period of months.

1961 — October. Three German physicians at a national meeting of gynecologists separately reported the appearance of large numbers of severely deformed babies wih a highly characteristic but hitherto extremely rare malformation termed *phocomelia* (Greek *phokos,* seal; *melia,* limbs), because of the flipper-like appearance of the legs and arms. These babies also often showed abnormalities of the heart and intestinal tract. About one-half of the infants died. The survivors were normally intelligent. At that time, no satisfactory explanation for this phenomenon was available; many possibilities were suspected.

1961 — November 18. At a meeting of West German pediatricians, Professor Lenz, one of the three physicians who had presented cases in October, told his colleagues of evidence indicating that thalidomide taken by the mother early in pregnancy might be the cause. (At about the same time, an Australian physician, McBride, independently arrived at the same conclusion.)

1961 — November 27. The producers of thalidomide, Chemie Grunenthal, withdrew the product under pressure from the press and the West German Ministry of Health. The Ministry issued a statement that the drug was suspected of being a major factor causing phocomelia. At the same time the firm Distillers, in

England, which sold thalidomide in the United Kingdom and the Commonwealth, voluntarily withdrew the drug, in view of the reports they had received of fetal deformities thought to be associated with the administration of the drug in early pregnancy. By this time, in the words of Professor Lenz, ". . . thousands of despaired and mourning parents were left with their dead or crippled children."

When the epidemic ended, Lenz estimated that between 6,000 and 8,000 cases had occurred in West Germany alone. Hundreds more were reported from many countries throughout the world.

Drug companies and health officials in other countries were slow to follow suit, despite widespread publicity. The last was Japan, where approximately 1,000 cases occurred. Withdrawal of the drug was completed there in January 1963 — more than one year after thalidomide was removed from the market in Germany. As Dr. Helen Taussig pointed out at that time, part of the lag resulted from the fact that thalidomide masqueraded in seventeen countries under close to a hundred trade names; part was obviously due to the reluctance of officials to take action which would antagonize drug companies and pharmacists; and part was due to reluctance of the drug houses to relinquish profits.

In each country, approximately nine months after thalidomide was withdrawn from sale, the epidemic ceased. The few cases appearing thereafter could be accounted for by the fact that tablets not returned had been consumed by pregnant women unaware of the danger.

The evidence that thalidomide produced phocomelia can be summarized as follows:

1. *Association.* When accurate information could be obtained, it was found that most of the mothers who gave birth to the deformed infants had taken some form of the drug early in pregnancy. (There was no relationship with the size of the dose.) Conversely, comparable groups of women who clearly had not taken thalidomide did not give birth to babies with the deformities. In addition, in each country where information was available, the volume of sales of the

drug closely parallelled the frequency of the malformations, with an expected time lag of about nine months. No other positive associations have been found.

2. *Timing.* The details of the sequence of the development of the human fetus within the uterus is well known to embryologists. Professor Lenz was able to show that knowledge of the time in days after the last menstrual period at which the pregnant woman took thalidomide allowed prediction of the type of resulting malformation. For example: deformities of the ears and cranial nerves correlated with an intake between the 34th and 38th days; absence of the arms indicated intake after the 39th day; absence of the gall bladder and abnormalities of the small intestine, together with malformation of the heart, related to intake between the 40th and 50th days. No malformation occurred when the drug was taken after the 50th day.

3. *Geography.* Only a few cases occurred in France, the United States, the East German Democratic Republic, and Czechoslovakia, where the drug had not been released for sale; those few could be attributed to tablets imported into the country by the mother, or used in clinical trials. Europe, Australia, Canada, South America, Africa and Japan were involved in this unique epidemic.

4. *Animal Experimentation.* After the disaster, malformations were produced by thalidomide in the offspring of rabbits and monkeys. In the pregnant monkey, a single dose given at the appropriate time caused malformations very like those in humans, in almost 100 per cent of the offspring. At the present time, a cause and effect relationship is accepted.

Could this tragedy have been prevented or mitigated? It is commonly assumed that it was unavoidable. Previously, few congenital malformations in babies had been attributed to drugs taken by the mother early in pregnancy. Most physicians were unaware that this can be a particularly vulnerable time. Testing of new drugs for possible teratogenic properties was not a standard procedure at that time. However, eight months before the effects of thalidomide were realized, the Committee on Fetus and Newborn of the American Academy of Pediatrics had specifically written a warning about the serious hazards to the fetus of drugs given to the mother. Lenz had pointed out that this was only one of a series of warnings which began appearing in 1955. Both in England and in Germany the drug was advertised as being perfectly safe during pregnancy. In addition, there was the problem of polyneuritis, which had been recognized and reported to Chemie Grunenthal in 1959. According to Sjostrom and Nilsson, the company had received reports of over a hundred cases of severe polyneuritis (an inflammation of the sensory nerves) at a time when only a handful of reports had appeared in the medical literature. By the time the drug was withdrawn, the number of cases of polyneuritis was approximately the same as the number of cases of phocomelia. Chemie Grunenthal continued to represent their product as completely harmless. In addition, they specifically recommended the drug for the treatment of nausea so common in early pregnancy. (By the end of May 1961 the number of reported cases of polyneuritis is said to have approximated 1,300.)

It is clear that the advertising and promotion of thalidomide in West Germany were totally irresponsible and misleading; it is almost certain that there was a cover-up of information available to the company.

The probability that this disaster could have been prevented or at least minimized is made more plausible by the well-known fact that it was deliberately prevented from occurrence in the United States because of concern about hazards of health. (Thalidomide was restricted from France and Czecholslovakia apparently for trade reasons.) This prevention in the United States was due largely to the vigilance of a stubborn, alert, intelligent woman, Dr. Frances Kelsey, who subsequently received a Presidential award for her efforts.

In September 1960 the Merrell Company applied to the United States' Federal Food and Drug Administration for registration of thalidomide, in order to market the drug. In doing so, they submitted detailed data and evidence regarding its properties. Dr. Kelsey, acting for the FDA, postponed acceptance, requesting more data concerning the toxicity. Her objections were threefold:

1. The appearance of a few reports of polyneuritis in patients taking the drug chronically.

2. The lack of complete data regarding the effect on animals of giving the drug for long periods of time (*i.e.*, at least one year).
3. The need for evidence that thalidomide did not damage the fetus when administered to mothers early in pregnancy. (This third objection stemmed from the first two. Also it appears to result from Dr. Kelsey's previous scientific work on teratogenic agents.)

In spite of considerable pressure from the Merrell Company, impatient because of repeated postponements and requests for more detailed information, the officials at the FDA held fast. In November 1961 the drug was removed from the market in Germany. In March of the following year, the Merrell Company withdrew its application.

The United States was not the only country to reject thalidomide on the basis that it might be a hazard to health. It was subsequently brought out in a Swedish court that the East German Democratic Republic had refused to admit the drug early in 1951 because of reports of toxicity to the nervous system and because of inadequate animal and human trials.

Following the total withdrawal of thalidomide from all countries, there has been an extensive series of court cases in most areas where phocomelia has occurred. Most of these resulted from lawsuits brought by associations of parents of the deformed children. Many millions of dollars have been expended by many drug companies, for the most part in out-of-court settlements.

Sjostrom, the co-author of the book, *Thalidomide and the Power of the Drug Companies,* and a lawyer representing the plaintiffs in many of the cases, tells the story. In Aachen, Germany, the public prosecutor initiated criminal proceedings against nine of the Chemie Grunenthal Associates. Documents of the company were seized in police raids. Many records had been destroyed. The disaster had been an international scandal resulting in world-wide attention to the long-drawn-out, bitter trials. The trial was suspended in 1970 after six years of preliminary investigation and two and a half years of courtroom proceedings — *not* because the Chemie Grunenthal Company was found guilty or not guilty, but rather because the court felt it was not in the public interest to pursue the matter further.

No errors of treatment have ever caused such changes in attitude or produced so much legislation in so many countries. In 1962, Dr. Helen Taussig expressed the feelings of thousands: "One sad story is, we hope, coming to an end. It should be the dawn of new and better control of drugs."

These effects and the lessons learned will be discussed in Chapter 5.

Another Reducing Pill — High Blood Pressure in the Lungs

An unusual and probably unpredictable epidemic was one appearing in central Europe in 1967 and 1968, in association with the use of a new drug, aminorex.

Among both doctors and the public the term *hypertension* is usually used to indicate a rise in blood pressure in the arteries which supply all of the body except the lungs. But a rare condition does exist in which an unexplained elevation of blood pressure occurs in the separate pulmonary arterial circuit without elevation of pressure in the systematic circuit (the arteries to the rest of the body). This rare condition is termed *primary pulmonary hypertension* and is due to changes in the very small arteries in the lungs, increasing the resistance to blood flow through them. The University Medical Clinic in Berne had for a decade averaged less than one admission a year of a patient with this disease until 1967, when Dr. Gurtner, a Swiss cardiologist, noted an impressive change. Adult patients, nearly all overweight, young or middle-aged, and mostly female began appearing in increasing numbers in the clinic, complaining of shortness of breath, tiring on exertion, fainting attacks, and occasional chest pains. The heart sounds, the chest x-rays, and the electrocardiograms all indicated that the right side of the heart, which pumps the blood through the lungs, was overloaded. Diagnostic heart catheterization tests, the only way of measuring pressure in the pulmonary arteries, indicated that the patients had primary pulmonary hypertension. Twenty-three cases appeared in a period of eighteen months. Similar increases were also found in other Swiss centres. In Germany and Austria, the epidemic started about a year later and was less marked.

Many things were considered and excluded as possible causes, including environmental agents such as dust, sprays, plastic substances and household chemicals. There was no evidence of an infectious process. Drugs were also suspected — particularly the oral contraceptives — and patients were closely questioned regarding their use, once the existence of an epidemic was recognized. The only medicine commonly used by most of these patients was aminorex, an appetite-depressing agent introduced on the Swiss market in November 1965. (Later it was sold in Germany and Austria.) Eighty per cent of the patients reported taking the medicine before developing symptoms. Analysis of information on a large number of persons who had taken aminorex showed a progressive increase in incidence of the disease with the number of tablets ingested. About 10 per cent of the women who had taken more than 360 tablets developed primary pulmonary hypertension.

Though the causal relationship between the disease and the drug was not considered proven, aminorex was taken off the Swiss market, and also the German and Austrian markets in October 1968, three years after its introduction. A joint study in six Swiss centres by the Swiss Society of Cardiology in 1970 discovered 308 cases proven by cardiac catheterization or autopsy between the years 1965 and 1970, with 26 deaths in this group. It was demonstrated that in Switzerland, the peak of the epidemic occurred in 1968 and 1969. New cases did not appear after 1970. Nearly all patients began having symptoms about nine months after beginning to take the drug. Unfortunately, the pulmonary hypertension in the surviving patients did not disappear or lessen when they discontinued aminorex.

Animal experiments, performed in the usual fashion before the drug was released for human use and again more searchingly after the epidemic, failed to produce the disease in dogs and rats. However, acute experiments injecting aminorex intravenously in dogs readily demonstrated high sustained pressures in the pulmonary arteries, and chronic feeding of the drug to rats also elevated these pressures. Proof of a causal association between the drug and the disease rests entirely on the strong epidemiological evidence of geography, timing in relation to sales, age, sex, and history of intake — also the disappearance of the epidemic on the withdrawal of aminorex from the market. The statistical probability is high that causal association does exist. Though there is no evidence that careful, long-term controlled clinical trials were made, the disease was quickly detected and dealt with.

Another Synthetic Hormone — Cancer of Vagina in Daughters

The alertness of a gynecologist and his colleagues, who recognized in 1971 the possibility of an epidemic after seeing only eight cases of a rare disease, led to the discovery of one of the most delayed and curious of all the drug side-effects.

Between 1966 and 1969, eight teen-age girls suffering from cancer of the vagina, were seen in one Boston gynecological clinic. The physicians, A. L. Herbst and his colleagues, recognized the unusual nature of the occurrence of such a cluster of cases. A review of the medical literature confirmed their suspicions. This group of females constituted a larger number of cases than had been previously reported altogether in this age group in the entire century.

This experience led to a systematic search for factors which might be associated with the appearance of these tumours. First, a check was made for similarities among the patients, with respect to habits, medication, and symptoms. Then four carefully matched controls were selected for each girl with cancer. The matching was made according to age (birth within five days of the patient); location (birth at the same hospital and on the same service, ward or private); and sex (female). The mothers of patients and controls were interviewed personally by a trained interviewer from a standard questionnaire. The factors considered included birth weight, maternal smoking habits, bleeding during pregnacy, previous miscarriages or abortions, specific hormonsal treatment during pregnancy, ingestion of other medications during pregnancy, breast feeding, exposure to x-ray during pregnancy, childhood diseases of patients and parents, and even household pets. Employing sophisticated analyses of these multiple factors, Herbst and his co-workers found "a highly significant association" between the treatment of the mothers with stilbestrol and the subsequent development of cancer of the vagina in their daughters "(p less than 0.00001)." (The "p less than 0.00001" is the statistician's way of expressing the fact that the likelihood of such an association's occurring by chance was less than one in a hundred thousand.) Other factors found to be associated but at lower levels of probability included bleeding during pregnancy, and previous abortions or miscarriages. These last two associations were easily explained by the fact that stilbestrol was given to the mothers in order to prevent bleeding and miscarriage. Thus, despite the fact that only eight patients with the disease were available, it was possible to discover a highly probable causal factor.

Additional information supplemented that derived from this ingenious epidemological approach. The patients were born between 1946 and 1953, at a time when stilbestrol was commonly being used to prevent threatened abortion. The drug was known to be capable of causing cancer in animals, and, under certain rare conditions, in man; but at the time few physicians were aware of the potential hazards of administering *any* drug to a pregnant woman.

Following the publication of the report from Boston, the FDA and the Australian Drug Evaluation Committee issued warnings against the use of stilbestrol in pregnancy.

Herbst and his group developed a registry by corresponding with their colleagues in many geographical areas. By December 1972 they had compiled a digest of ninety-one cases reporting adenocarcinoma of the vagina in females between the ages of eight and twenty-five. Information was available regarding the medication used during the pregnancy of the mother in sixty-six cases.. Forty-nine of these mothers had received stilbestrol.

This delay of the appearance of a toxic side-effect for thirteen to twenty-two years, similar to the delay in the appearance of carcinoma of the thyroid in the adolescents irradiated by x-ray during infancy, opened up new possibilities not previously anticipated, and clearly established another drug as a carcinogen.

CHAPTER FOUR

Overdose

In contrast to drugs which are no longer used because of their toxic side effects, there are useful drugs with side effects caused by overdose. They are now given with moderation and caution. In each instance, widespread suffering and often death occurred over a period of years before the nature of the problem was recognized and corrected.

In this chapter we see how overdose and abuse of oxygen were followed by blindness; of vitamin D, by poisoning; of an inhalant for the relief of asthmatic attacks, by sudden unexpected death; of a commonly used remedy for diarrhea, by paralysis; of a useful headache remedy, by severe damage to the kidneys.

Oxygen — and an Epidemic of Blindness in Premature Infants

One of the most devastating of the results of overdose of a drug was that occurring as a result of the use of excessive amounts of oxygen.

In the late thirties, pediatricians and ophthalmologists in the United States began to notice a peculiar form of blindness in babies. Attention was called to it in a classic report by Theodore Terry, a professor of ophthalmology at Harvard, who recognized that it was a condition not previously described and that it occurred only in infants born prematurely. Terry labelled it "retrolental fibroplasia (RLF)," because the abnormality appeared to consist of an overgrowth of fibrous tissue behind the lens of the eyes. Later it was learned that RLF was really a disease of the developing retina, which often became detached.)

Soon after this first recognition, many cases were reported confirming the original findings. Within a few years it became the largest single cause of blindness in the United States. Almost a fourth of premature infants weighing less than four pounds at birth were afflicted. By 1950 it had become a world-wide problem involving thousands. Epidemiologically it was a strange disease, varying greatly in frequency among cities (at first common in Boston, but absent in Baltimore), and also even among the nurseries in the hospitals of each city. Often no cases were observed in one premature nursery, while in another a mile or two away, the disease was common.

For years there was speculation as to the origin of this new epidemic. It seemed unlikely that it was a congenital malformation, since the disease developed between two and six months after birth. Three years after his original description, Terry listed possible causes: heredity, infection within the eye, precocious exposure to daylight, an increase or decrease of oxygen in the blood, the lower temperature of the premature babies in the incubator in contrast to the temperature of the fetus within the uterus before birth, inability to digest food or vitamins, birth trauma. He was inclined to favour precocious exposure to light as the most likely. Many other possibilities were added within the next few years, including sulfanilamide and antibiotic treatment, hormonal deficiency, vitamin B deficiency, the solvent in which vitamins administered were dissolved, iron medication, and excess vitamin A. Most of these leads were investigated without success, except for vitamin E and increase of oxygen.

Then, in 1951 several physicians independently came to the conclusion that the only common factor was related to the use of oxygen, some believing that its abrupt withdrawal after the premature infant was exposed to a high concentration was the cause; others felt that it was the high concentraion of oxygen per se which was responsible. Kate Campbell, a pediatrician in Australia, learning of this debate, reviewed the incidence of RLF in the nurseries of three Melbourne hospitals under her care, the management in which was the same except for the amount of oxygen used. In the first institution, oxygen was piped and given freely at a level of 40 to 60 per cent (air contains 21 per cent oxygen). In the second nursery, oxygen had to be given by funnel, and the concentration was less. In the third, in which only private patients were kept, cost was a consideration, and oxygen was given intermittently and in lowest concentration. No cases of retrolental fibroplasia had been observed in any of these institutions in 1946 and 1947. During the three years 1948, 1949, and 1950, at the first institution, 23 out of 123 premature infants developed RLF; 3 out of 44 at the second; and only 1 of 14 at the third. While this was only a retrospective report with no concurrent controls, it provided the first clinical data to associate RLF strongly with the use of high concentrations of oxygen. The use of oxygen in those Melbourne nurseries was then restricted to emergencies, and no further cases of blindness occurred in premature infants born there.

Some observers confirmed Campbell's experience, but others could not. In the fall of 1952, another opthalmologist, Arnall Patz, and his co-workers at Johns Hopkins reported a planned concurrent controlled study placing premature infants on either a high or a low oxygen routine, on a random basis. At the end of a year, seven of twenty-eight infants in the high oxygen had advanced RLF, while no cases of severe RLF occurred in the thirty-seven infants in the low oxygen group.

At the same institution before Patz did his study, a careful controlled clinical trial was conducted, evaluating the use of vitamin E. The results were most encouraging in that there occurred substantially less blindness among the Vitamin E treated premature infants as compared to the controls. The babies were all observed in the same nursery, and except for the administration of the vitamin, were said to have been given identical care. This new tested treatment was widely accepted and used for a short time. Unfortunately, at other centres, the pediatricians did not find that the vitamin E protected the babies. Later, when the importance of the high oxygen concentration was known, it was possible to account for the early apparent partial success with vitamin E. For obvious reasons, no placebo had been used. In order to give the vitamin to the treated group, it was necessary to open the incubators widely several times every 24 hours, thereby decreasing substantially the concentration of oxygen this group inhaled. This was an unusual example of the importance during a controlled clinical trial of making sure that both the specifically treated and the control groups receive the same care in every respect, except for the remedy being tested. Attention to small details is essential in the performance of these evaluations.

At first the data implicating high concentrations of oxygen were not widely accepted, but others, including reports of investigators in a large co-operative study involving eighteen participating hospitals in the United States in 1955, confirmed that the length of time the premature infant was kept in an oxygen-enriched environment determined the likelihood of the development of RLF.

Much of the reluctance to accept oxygen as the toxic agent related to the strong feelings on the part of clinicians to regard oxygn as harmless — after all, it is the stuff we breathe. Paul Bert, a famous French physiologist, in the last century had demonstrated toxic effects of very high oxygen concentrations on the lungs of adult animals, but the eyes had not been damaged.

In 1952 two Swedish investigators in Stockholm exposed newborn mice* to 100 per cent oxygen intermittently for periods of one to three weeks. These clinicians clearly demonstrated a specific destructive effect on the growing blood vessels in the retina, with subsequent detachment. The results were quickly confirmed by other workers in England and in the United States with tests on kittens and puppies. In addition, it was shown that obliteration of blood vessels in the retina was directly proportioned to the degree of immaturity of the retina, to the duration of exposure to oxygen, and to the degree of oxygen concentration.

By 1955 there was wide acceptance of the clinical evidence and the results of animal tests. Except for unusual circumstances in which high concentrations of oxygen were thought to be essential for life, the use of oxygen was restricted to levels of 35 to 40 per cent. This level was found to have no effect on animal newborns even after prolonged exposure. Subsequently it became clear that it was the tension of oxygen in the arterial blood which was important, *not,* directly, the concentration inhaled. This fact permits the use of extra oxygen in the treatment of pneumonia and other lung

---

*Newborn mice, kittens, and other species have at birth a development of the retina comparable to that of the newborn infant.

diseases in order to restore the level in the arterial blood to normal, but not above it.

These changes in treatment resulted in the dramatic disappearance of the disease — a devastating world-wide epidemic of permanent blindness caused by an overdosage of one of the most common and seemingly harmless substances. The production of the overdose was the result of advances in technology — piped-in oxygen and efficient incubators — one of the many instances in which technology advanced faster than the effects of its application.

Vitamin D — High Blood Calcium

Unlike the overdoses of the other drugs discussed in this chapter, the excessive use of vitamin D has occurred under rather different circumstances, leading to different conditions.

Rickets, the bone-deforming disease of children born in the winter months to city dwellers of Europe, has been known for centuries. The typical deformities can be seen in the child in some of the Nativity scenes by German and Dutch painters of the 15th century. At the beginning of the present century, it was considered by many to be an infectious disease. It was common in all northern industrial areas; between one-half and three-fourths of all infants were affected. Weakened by the disease, many died of infections. By 1930 a series of investigations had established the cause, cure, and prevention of this crippling deficiency disease. Vitamin D in its various forms, found naturally in cod liver, in the skin exposed to the ultraviolet rays of sunlight, or synthesized in the biochemist's laboratory, cured rickets. The discovery and the use of this vitamin was one of the outstanding accomplishments of preventive medicine; rickets is rarely seen today.

However, the misuse and overdose of this drug have led to two special problems: the production of serious damage to the kidney by the administration of massive daily doses for the treatment of disease other than rickets; and the occurrence of elevated blood calcium levels — hypercalcemia — and illness in normal infants given excessive vitamin D supplements in their food. Under suspicion is the role of too much vitamin D given during pregnancy in the abnormal development of the arteries, together with mental retardation and "elfin-like" facial appearances in infants and children born of the mothers.

Because vitamins are naturally present in food or are formed in the body, and because they are necessary for the growth, development, and well-being of the body, there has been a belief on the part of the public and many doctors that vitamins can do only good. They are usually not considered drugs or medicines. In spite of a complete lack of evidence that more than the usual requirements are an advantage, many millions of dollars are wasted in this country and in Great Britain on vitamin preparations of all varieties. It is true that the range between the ordinary therapeutic dose and that which causes harm is generally wide for vitamin D, but it has been known since 1928 that a massive dose could be toxic to animals and humans. Nevertheless, many clinicians continued to prescribe large doses for long periods of time to patients with hay fever, tuberculosis, psoriasis, and other chronic skin diseases. The treatment of tuberculosis in children with large doses of vitamin D was based on the experience in the 19th century of French clinicians who claimed good results in using huge amounts of cod liver oil for periods up to six months. Many individual cases of the above-mentioned maladies were said to be improved following this treatment, though its value was never established. In addition, some food faddists consumed large amounts for months or years. Numbers of highly concentrated preparations became available for sale without prescription. Part of the problem lay in the great variation existing in individual susceptibility to the toxic action of vitamin D. Some individuals are able to tolerate doses 900 times larger than the ordinary dose used for treating vitamin D deficiency; others develop symptoms when given several times the usual maintenance dose. Because most persons could tolerate the very large doses, many physicians felt confident in using them. In addition, there was in adults the safety feature usually manifested in symptoms such as loss of appetite, headache, nausea and vomiting, permitting withdrawal of the drug before the characteristic damage to the kidneys occurred.

Between 1940 and 1960, a series of cases of damage to kidneys with calcification, with a number of fatalities, was reported. Though no controlled studies were conducted, by 1960 experts were agreed that the vitamin D treatment of tuberculosis, psoriasis, and rheumatoid arthritis was both hazardous and ineffective.

A second manifestation of an overdose of vitamin D is a condition first recognized in 1952 by an observant pediatrician named Lightwood at the Hospital for Sick Children in London. In pediatrics, "failure to thrive" is a commonly used euphemism for complete failure to grow and develop in any fashion approaching normal. There are, of course, many causes. Lightwood observed several infants in a short period of time, all of whom suffered loss of appetite, vomiting, constipation, weakness, failure to thrive, and in addition an elevated level of calcium in the blood (hypercalcemia). All of the babies were receiving cow's milk, which contains much more calcium than does breast milk. Even though the individual intake of vitamin D was well below those which were considered toxic levels, it was several times greater than the minimal requirements of 400 units daily for prevention of rickets in the normal infant. Characteristically, the babies spontaneously recovered, after several months of illness, when the calcium and the vitamin D intake were reduced.

During the following two years the British Pediatric Association was able to secure reports on 216 confirmed cases of this form of infantile hypercalcemia from consultant pediatricians all over Great Britain. This number was in noticeable contrast to the rarity of the condition in the United States. Since the symptoms clinically and biochemically mimicked so closely the well-recognized intoxication with vitamin D seen in children and adults given huge doses, an overdose was suspected. From Finland a group of infants was reported with hypercalcemia and other findings similar in every way to the British cases. The Finnish babies had received large amounts of vitamin D by injection as part of the treatment for a refractory form of pneumonia.

Concerned about what appeared to be a true epidemic, and upon the advice of both the Medical Research Council and the British Pediatric Society, the Ministry of Health substantially reduced the allowances of vitamin D to about one-half the previous abount, *i.e.,* from 700 to 1,000 units to approximately the American standard of 400 units, and discontinued the free supplements of cod liver oil and of cereals and other foods enriched by vitamin D provided by the Infant Welfare Service. It was realized that this step might lead to a reduction of the margin of safety against rickets. By 1961 the incidence of hypercalcemia in Great Britain was less than half that reported in 1953, with no increase in the numbers of cases of rickets. The epidemic was over and has not recurred.

What appeared at first to be a third form of illness due to an excess of vitamin D was described in 1952 by the famous Swiss pediatrician Fanconi. The disease is characterized by permanent involvement of the brain, kidneys, arteries, and bones, as well as by hypercalcemia. A variable degree of mental retardation is present, and there is often a heart murmur; also, the children have an "elfin-like" facial appearance, making them easy to recognize. Since Fanconi's original description, two developments have occurred. First, further observations revealed many graduations between the mild and the severe forms of hypercalcemia. Second, two English pediatricians, Black and Bonham-Carter, noted the peculiar elfin-like face closely resembled that of children with a third condition called the supravalvar aortic stenosis (obstruction above the valve of the aorta) syndrome. More recently, two American physicians, Friedman and Roberts, have been able to produce very similar findings of both conditions, supravalvar aortic stenosis, and facial and dental changes in baby rabbits, by feeding the mother tremendous doses of vitamin D during the entire pregnancy. While many questions remain unanswered at the present time, it appears that these conditions — Lightwood's disease, Fanconi's disease, and supravalvar aortic stenosis — are related conditions. It is accepted that vitamin D plays an important role in their production. The reason that some infants are hypersensitive to this drug and respond abnormally remains obscure.

Vitamin D is not the only vitamin causing illness when given in excess. Large amounts of vitamin A administered to infants and children will produce a peculiar disease manifested by malaise, growth failure, changes in growing bone, and sometimes increased pressure within the skull. Recovery follows reduction of the dose.

These foregoing facts have served to remind all physicians that vitamins are potent drugs with special hazards, when used in medicinal form. When employed as food supplements, they require caution — particularly during infancy and pregnancy.

Another Headache Powder — an Epidemic of Kidney Disease

One of the most puzzling as well as one of the largest of the epidemics produced by overdose and abuse of drugs is kidney disease associated with the use of phenacetin-containing compounds. Along with the laxatives and vitamins, mild pain relievers and headache remedies are the most widely over-used drugs. An American novelist has described the present era as the "Aspirin Age." Millions of people do not let a day go by without taking medication of this type for prevention of symptoms as well as for relief of symptoms. Aspirin alone is most commonly used, and many suffer from its abuse; but, on the whole, its usefulness and effectiveness are considered to outweigh the harmful results.

Such does not appear to be the case with respect to the related synthetic chemical, phenacetin, also called acetaphenetidin. The commonly used combination called APC is a mixture of phenacetin with aspirin and caffeine, but phenacetin alone is seldom used. In combination with other drugs, it is sold under many trade names.

Though it had been on the market for three-quarters of a century, it was not until 1953 that the association between the use of phenacetin and an increasing number of cases of kidney disease became suspected in Europe — particularly in Germany, Switzerland, Scandinavia, and Czechoslovakia. Later, cases were recognized in Australia. Numbers of persons, with a particular type of chronic kidney disease of unknown cause, were found with a history of ingestion of large amounts of pain-relieving mixtures, all of which contained phenacetin — up to 100 to 150 tablets weekly for many years. Until the association between the disease and the drug was suspected, most patients failed on routine questioning to give a history of chronic use of this medicine, because they regarded it as a household remedy not worth special mention. Large numbers of supposedly healthy people in European countries were in the habit of regularly consuming large quantities of phenacetin-containing compounds, claiming they felt better and were able to work more efficiently as a result. The first reports of side effects came from Switzerland, where a mixture containing caffeine, aminopyrine (another pain reliever), and phenacetin, called by the trade name Saridon, was used. The patients were mostly women working in watch factories. Because they complained that the meticulous, close work gave them eye strain and headaches, bowls of tablets were made freely available to them, on the work tables. Subsequently, a series of reports, mostly from Scandinavian countries, appeared, with the same story of chronic kidney disease in factory workers who used phenacetin daily.

Altogether over 2,000 cases have been reported from Europe, over 100 from the United States, and 45 from Canada. Several hundred patients have died from chronic kidney failure. The symptoms, excluding those for which the paient was taking the pain-relieving compound, included malaise, weakness, vomiting, loss of weight, and often pains in the flank, together with blood in the urine. Because of the flank pain, the patients often increased their dose of pain killers, thus almost surely further damaging their kidneys.

Several facts indicate that the relationship between this particular form of kidney disease and phenacetin itself is not that of a simple cause and effect. First, it has not been possible to satisfactorily duplicate the disease in animals, using phenacetin alone, though combinations, such as APC, will produce similar changes when given for periods of many months. Aspirin taken for long periods can produce damage to the kidneys in both animals and man. However, many of the preparations used did not contain aspirin; phenacetin was the only chemical common to all. Second, there were no good control or comparison data. (A study is in progress at the present time.) Third, the true incidence of this form of kidney disease was not known before the initial reports. The apparent increase in the numbers of cases may have been due to the fact that they were looked for more energetically and with better diagnostic facilities; the diagnosis was simply made more often.

On the other hand, the epidemiologic and circumstantial evidence was strong. The geographic location of the cases corresponded well with sale and habits of abuse of this form of analgesic in the countries involved, by factory workers and older persons troubled by headaches or chronic pains. Relatively few cases have been reported from England, the United States, and Canada, where the habits of the factory workers are not the same. That most patients were female could be explained by the fact that the medication was commonly taken to relieve menstrual cramps or symptoms of the menopause.

On the other hand, a recent study from a county hospital in Sweden points out that there were more men than women with this illness. Between 1954 and 1970 at that institution, 116 persons who were abusers of phenacetin died of unexplained kidney failure; only 25 of them were women. In this instance, the ratio could be due to the fact that 60 of the men worked at one factory employing only men.

The most significant piece of evidence has been the gratifying decrease in the numbers of cases since the sale of phenacetin-containing preparations was sharply restricted. The drug became subject either to prescription or withdrawal from compounds in Switzerland, Sweden, and Denmark. Following such restriction, in 1961 in Sweden the consumption of phenacetin declined tenfold. The percentage of cases among chronic users of pain-relieving medication dropped from 58 per cent in 1961 to 25 per cent in 1965. In the same Swedish county hospital mentioned above, the numbers of deaths increased until 1966; then sharply fell off in 1970. This lag can be explained by the assumption based on clinical evidence that even if the drug is stopped, death from kidney failure may occur as long as eight years later. In western Scotland, where phenacetin was withdrawn from Asket Powders and Beecham's Powders in 1966 (two much-used proprietary preparations), the numbers of new cases diagnosed as analgesic nephropathy seen in one large kidney clinic in Glasgow remained fairly constant until 1971, when they dropped sharply. A similar experience has been reported from Denmark; the exception has been Australia. There, paracetamol, a drug similar to phenacetin, has been substituted for phenacetin. Until now there has been little change in the incidence of new cases.

A related disturbing recent development has been the appearance of a number of individual case reports suggesting an association between the development of cancer of the bladder or kidney and the excessive use of phenacetin.

It is surprising and discouraging that this useful but non-essential drug could have been in widespread general use for over forty years before its ill effects were recognized. In this respect, this error is unique. The lesson appears to lie in the hazards inherent in the unrestricted widespread use of potent but non-essential remedies.

A Diarrhea Remedy — Paralysis

What appears to have been the longest and largest epidemic associated with a common drug is the outbreak of a strange disease resembling a form of encephalitis, which began in Japan in 1956 and extended through the 1960s. It followed the over-use of clioquinol — known in most western countries as Entero-Vioform.

In the second half of the 1950s, Japanese doctors began seeing patients with an unusual chronic disorder manifested by adbominal pains and diarrhea, followed by neurological disturbances and occasionally by death. A chronic relapsing disease often lasting years, it was unlike anything previously seen in Japan or other countries. The neurological disturbances consisted of numbness, tingling, coldness, and weakness of the feet, these symptoms tending to progress gradually upward with some degree of paralysis in about half the patients. About one in four developed some trouble with vision, complete blindness occurring on rare occasions. Slightly over half the patients recovered after a long illness; approximately one in twenty died.

The numbers of cases irregularly increased with sporadic outbreaks as the years went by, until, at the peak of the epidemic in 1969, 300 new cases were seen in one month. At the annual meeting of the Japanese Society of Internal Medicine in 1965, it was generally agreed that this was an entirely new clinical entity of unknown cause — a major health problem. The term *subacute myelo-optico neuropathy* (abbreviated to SMON) was adopted because of 1) the subacute onset of the disease, and 2) the neurological changes involving the peripheral nerves, spinal cord, and optic nerves. The term SMON is now widely used because of its obvious brevity and convenience.

In 1967, alarmed by two recent outbreaks, the Ministry of Health organized and financed a large special SMON research commission to study the epidemiology of the disease, the possible causes, and to find effective therapeutic and preventive measures. The sixty-four members of this commission included epidemiologists, micro-biologists, clinicians, neurologists, neuro-pathologists, and pharmocologists — one of the largest groups of experts ever assembled to study a single epidemic. In spite of all this activity, few outside Japan knew of SMON until the last few years. At that time, it was known to exist only in Japan, and nearly all of the many publications were in Japanese.

For years SMON was thought to be an encephalitis due to an infection, but most of the epidemiological evidence emerging did not support the earlier view. In favour of arguments supporting the theories that the epidemic was of an infectious nature were the following chacteristics:

1. The endemic occurrence of the disease in small cities and towns for several years, followed by disappearance.
2. Outbreaks in families, clinics, or hospitals.
2. The apparent increased exposure to the disease of doctors, nurses, and medical technicians.
4. The seasonal prevalence in the summer.
5. The lack of relationship with industry or trades, such as mining or fishing.

Against the theory that the disease was of an infectious nature were the following facts:

1. SMON was a new disease, at first localized in Japan.
2. It was rare in children and common among middle-aged or older women.
3. In most areas it was sporadic, and contact cases were difficult to trace.
4. The clinical course of the disease did not suggest an infection. There was neither fever nor rash; the blood and spinal

fluid showed none of the abnormalities usually present in encephalitis.

5. The microscopic examination of nerve tissue removed from patients at autopsy did not suggest an infectious process.

Repeated efforts were made to isolate a virus. One group of investigators claimed to have succeeded in discovering one in the stool and spinal fluid of patients which could produce similar changes when injected into the brains of mice. They also found evidence for the presence of a virus from special immunochemical tests. However, the scientists at the Central Virus Diagnostic Laboratory at the National Institute of Health in Tokyo were unable to confirm these results. In addition, they believed that the pathologic changes in the nervous systems of the injected mice were dissimilar in distribution and type to those occurring in patients dying of SMON.

Other possibilities — the pesticides (more used in Japan than in any other country), industrial poisons such as mercury, food additives, and vitamin deficiencies secondary to malabsorption from the intestinal tract produced by an infection — were all considered and excluded. Furthermore, special bacteriological studies of the bacterial flora of the intestinal tract failed to show important differences in patients as compared to controls.

Medications were also suspected, of course, but no drug was strongly implicated until 1970. In February of that year, the clinical observation was made that some patients had a greenish "fur" on their tongues, which was at first thought to be the result of infection. A few months later, green discolouration of the urine and feces was noted, and chemical analyses were performed. These identified the green pigment as the molecule of the drug known as clioquinol, bound to iron. Later, the pigment was also identified by gas chromatography as clioquinol.

The history of this well-known and widely used drug is an interesting one. It is an organic iodide — iodochlorohydroxyquinoline — with more than fifty trade names, sold in many countries and known in the western world most often as Entero-Vioform. It was introduced in 1933 and was at first used for the treatment of amoebic dysentery; since then it has become popular in most countries around the world for the prevention of travellers' diarrhea, with the reputation of being one of the least toxic of effective drugs because of its apparent poor absorption from the intestinal tract. In Japan this drug was incorporated into 184 types of proprietary remedies sold over the counter and known as "sei-cho-zai," roughly translated as medicines "active in normalizing intestinal function." Millions consumed these medications for vague intestinal complaints for long periods of time — months or years — both with and without medical advice. (In western countries, the drug is seldom taken for more than a week or two.)

The following year (1971), Tsubaki, a neurologist, and his associates energetically pursued the hypothesis that SMON was caused by clioquinol. A detailed survey with careful questioning in seven hospitals revealed the following:

1. 96 per cent of 171 patients with the disease had taken the clioquinol before neurological symptoms appeared; no other drug was strongly associated.
2. The onset of symptoms corresponded with specific amounts of medication, usually several hundred grams over a period of one to four months.
3. Large doses tended to be associated with more severe illness.
4. Hospitalized patients with intestinal disorders who had not received clioquinol did not develop SMON.

The results seemed to indicate an attack rate of about 3 to 10 per cent of those using the drug for prolonged periods.

With the available initial information, the Ministry of Health and Welfare in the fall of 1970 prohibited the sale of clioquinol and warned doctors and the general public not to use preparations containing this drug. In addition, the World Health Organization was notified, and it in turn communicated the information to member countries. Thereafter an abrupt, sharp decrease followed in the numbers of new cases seen each month. In all of 1972 only a few new cases were reported in spite of continuous nationwide surveillance.

In addition to this strong circumstantial epidemiological evidence, animal experiments on rats, hamsters, rabbits, and dogs demonstrated clioquinol to be toxic to nerves and the spinal cord.

The pathologic damage in dogs and rabbits closely mimicked that seen in human cases of SMON.

One of the puzzles was the fact that the disease was largely limited to Japan. A difference in genetic constitution was suggested. However, recently cases have been reported from Australia, France, and the Netherlands, where the disease followed over-use of clioquinol in patients not of Japanese descent.

Still, in 1973 some qualified investigators in Japan continued to believe that an infectious process has not been excluded. One group in Tokyo believed that they had isolated a virus associated with SMON and argued that antibodies to the virus were formed in reaction to the disease. Other virologists have not found support for a viral cause. It is possible that a virus and clioquinol act in combination.

After the disease appeared in Australia in 1971 the government required that clioquinal be sold by prescription only. The British Committee of Safety of Medicines in 1973 reviewed the evidence and suggested that some other local factor must have acted synergistically with the drug. The Committee did not withdraw it from the market. They advised — and CIBA, the company involved, agreed — that warning should be included on all medicines containing clioquinol to the effect that they should not be taken for any prolonged period. The American editor of the 1973 *Yearbook of Drug Therapy* has suggested that this drug not be used until more is learned about why certain patients suffer toxic effects, and the American Center for Disease Control warned against its use for travelers' diarrhea. It is now sold in the U.S.A. under prescription only, for treatment of amoebic dysentery.

At present it appears that, like the kidney damage associated with phenacetin, SMON was the result of the drug-taking habits of the Japanese. The gross abuse of this non-essential drug by doctors and public alike produced disease and disability in more than 10,000 persons, and caused the deaths of several hundred. The epidemic lasted fifteen years.

An Inhalant for Asthma — Sudden Death

The most devastating epidemic following the excessive use of medication appears to have been the sudden unexpected deaths which resulted from the use of pressurized aerosol inhalers in the 1960s. It is likely that 3,500 deaths in the United Kingdom alone resulted from this form of symptomatic treatment, yet it went unsuspected for five years. (More deaths occurred in other countries.)

Bronchial asthma is an allergic disease in which, during the characteristic attacks, the airways into the lungs (the bronchi), go into spasm, causing the wheezing and shortness of breath so distressing and frightening to the patient; between attacks, he is often well. It has been known for many years that, while death may occur during an asthmatic attack, it is rare before middle age. Since cure can seldom be achieved, symptomatic treatment of the attacks is one of the important ways of giving relief. For many years, adrenalin given by injection has been known to relax the spasm of the bronchi and alleviate the distress. More recently, similar drugs with more rapid and effective action have been used, the most common being isoproterenol, at first administered by dissolving a tablet under the tongue. With the development of pressurized aerosol inhalants, it was found that adrenalin, isoproterenol, and other closely related drugs could be given in this simple fashion. The doses were metered and self-administered by the patient to relieve his attack.

Recognition of the problem began in 1964, when a physician in Australia reported sudden unexpected deaths in three asthmatic patients who had received isoproterenol by inhalation, followed by injections of adrenalin. The doctor ascribed the deaths to the combination of agents. This report was followed by a warning by the Australian Minister of Health against careless self-administration of inhalants and against a combination of these two drugs. The following year in a letter to *The Lancet,* Dr. Greenberg, a chest physician practicing in Cambridge, England, described how, in a period of eighteen months, eight of his asthmatic patients had died suddenly, following the excessive use of aerosol inhalers. Two other patients, one of whom had a severe cardiac arrhythmia, became pulseless. Dr. Greenberg believed that the deaths were cardiac rather than respiratory in nature and ascribed them to the effect of the drugs on the heart. In contrast to the Australian report, only half of his patients were given injections of adrenalin as well as the inhalant.

In 1966 Dr. Beryl Corner, an outstanding English pediatrician, presented a paper to a meeting of chest physicians which stimulated a careful epidemiological investigation of the whole problem. Dr. Corner analyzed the deaths of asthmatic children in the area around Bristol and found that there had been a substantial, unexplained increase between 1963 and 1966. This led to a large-scale national review of the situation. It was learned that the mortality attributed to asthma in England and Wales had steadily increased between 1960 and 1965, and that the increase was sevenfold in children between ten and fourteen years of age. This made asthma the fourth commonest cause of death in children in this age group. There was no immediate obvious explanation. No reason could be found to suspect changes in diagnosis or classification, nor did geographical distribution of the deaths implicate environmental factors. That mortality in all age groups was higher in the summer indicated the unimportance of epidemic respiratory infections; furthermore, there had been no apparent increase in the numbers of patients with asthma, but an increase in the numbers of deaths.

The only two common types of drugs used by persons who had died were cortisone and its related compounds (the steroids), and isoproterenol and similar bronchodilators in the form of pressurized aerosol inhalants. About one-third of the patients had been receiving steroids, while more than four-fifths were known to have used pressurized aerosols.

Cortisone and similar steroid drugs are commonly used to suppress allergic responses and thereby prevent attacks. Most often they are administered daily. Greenberg and his colleague, Pines, in a second letter to *The Lancet* in 1967 warned, "We suspect that patients with asthma may be killing themselves by the excessive use of sympathomimetic agents in the form of metered or pressurized aerosols containing isoprenaline, orciprenaline or adrenaline." Field workers of the English Committee on Safety of Drugs established strong circumstantial evidence of excessive use of the inhalers in many cases. In some instances the aerosol can was found by the patient's side or in his hand, for death often occurred outside the hospital. Reasons for over-use were obvious. The inhalant of the aerosol bronchodilators usually brings quick relief by reducing the resistance to the flow of air into the lung. However, it has long been known that with much use of these drugs, some patients become refractory and fail to respond. They are then inclined to try repeated doses in the attempt to obtain relief. A plausible explanation of the mechanism of sudden death was a severe disturbance of cardiac rhythm — ventricular tachycardia proceeding to ventricular fibrillation. The effect of isoproterenol on the heart has been known for years.

In June 1967 the Committee on Safety of Drugs sent a pamphlet to all doctors in the United Kingdom warning of possible hazards of these inhalants when used to excess. Six months later, they were still being sold, but by prescription only. In addition, the dangers were publicized widely.

Thereafter there was a gratifying decline in the numbers of fatalities; however, this trend had commenced at the end of 1965. Careful estimates of annual direct sales and prescriptions of each brand of inhaler were made. The numbers of deaths attributed to asthma in persons aged five to thirty-four years in England and Wales began increasing in 1961 and continued to rise to a peak in 1965 and 1966. By early 1967 there was a sharp fall in mortality, which continued in 1968 and 1969. The curve at the end of the the decade had almost reached the baseline of 1959 and 1960. Similarly, there had been a roughly parallel rise and fall in the total sales of pressurized aerosols. After reaching their highest level at the end of 1966 the sales levelled off for a year, then began to fall sharply. Both strong and weak preparations of isoproterenol had shown roughly the same pattern of rise and decline. Inman and Adelstein, reporting for the Committee on Safety of Drugs in London, stated in 1969: "The increase in mortality and in hospital admissions coincided with the growth of the use of pressurized aerosols. Between 1961 and 1967, there was at all ages a total of more than 3,500 deaths from asthma in excess of the number that would have been expected on the basis of experience of the two years (1959 and 1960) that preceded their use on a large scale . . . the ratio of deaths to aerosols used was similar in all age groups over five years."

Since then, Paul Stolley, an associate professor of epidemiology at Johns Hopkins University Medical School, in a controversial article entitled, "Why the United States was Spared an Epidemic of Deaths Due to Asthma," examined the problem from a global point of view. During the sixties, less marked unexplained increases in asthma mortality were also observed in Australia, New Zealand, Ireland, and several European countries; no increases occurred in the United States and Canada in spite of the fact that there had been a large sale of similar aerosol vapourizers in both countries. Stolley proposed the explanation that the high concentration of isoproterenol in 30 per cent of the aerosols sold in the United Kingdom might account for this difference. There the widely used nebulizers delivered five times the amount per spray than that licensed for use in the United States and Canada. He further argued, "Because it had been postulated that over-use of these nebulizers might lead to unexpected sudden death in asthmatics, a nebulizer five times more potent seems to present special hazards." Further investigation showed that in all of the countries with a marked rise in asthma mortality, the nebulizer containing the stronger concentration of isoproterenol was sold. However, in two countries where it was marketed, the Netherlands and Belgium, there was no increase in the number of asthma deaths. Stolley explained this discrepancy by the fact that the stronger preparation was not introduced into these countries until 1966, and that the sales per capita had been low. Stolley's conclusion was much more conservative than his title: "The evidence does not suggest that this highly concentrated isoproterenol preparation was the sole cause of the increased mortality; rather, it might have contributed to the severity of the epidemic of asthma mortality in countries in which the preparation was widely used." Some remain sceptical of this particular hypothesis. Inman and Doll found no selective relationship between mortality and the sales of the weaker preparations, as compared to the strong. (There was a closer association between deaths from asthma and direct sales of aerosols than between deaths from asthma sales on National Health Service prescriptions.) In Australia, where there had been a serious epidemic, no relation could be found between the sales of nebulizers and mortality in asthmatics.

Additional circumstantial evidence exists from animal trials. Tests on dogs demonstrated that in the presence of low oxygen concentrations in their arterial blood (as often occurs during asthmatic attack in humans), isoproterenol will produce a fall in blood pressure, followed by cardiac arrest. When the dogs were breathing room air and their arterial oxygen concentration was normal, the drug caused no ill effects.

At present, the hypothesis that the epidemic of sudden deaths in asthmatic patients in England and Wales in the 1960s was due to the over-use and abuse of the pressurized aerosol bronchodilators, chiefly isoproterenol, appears to be highly probable and is generally accepted. The epidemiological data of a causal association are strong, though not entirely consistent. Finally, after the most careful consideration and search, there has been no satisfactory alternative explanation for this devastating epidemic.

CHAPTER FIVE

Possible Errors — Not Proven

Throughout Man's history, hundreds of medical treatments, the value of which have never been proven or disproven, have come and gone. Most often they were replaced by new remedies thought at the time to be superior. The present century is no exception. Today there are many forms of therapy, medical and surgical, whose value remains in doubt.

In this section, four recent examples are considered, because they illustrate so well the need for carefully planned, controlled, clinical trials, in order that errors may not be perpetuated. The first of these, sympathectomy for high blood pressure, was a major surgical procedure; the second, a useful but presumably toxic pain reliever; the third, a treatment for heart attacks; the fourth, a drug to prevent migraine attacks.

Removal of the Sympathetic Nerves for High Blood Pressure

This operation, termed sympathectomy, was introduced in the 1930s, performed on thousands of patients, and largely given up in the 1960s because of the introduction of effective medical treatment. The value of the surgery was never properly tested and is still in doubt.

High blood pressure — chronic elevation of the pressure in the arterial system without apparent specific cause (essential hypertension) — is one of the most common of all chronic diseases and a major cause of death in modern society. The elevation of pressure is produced by increased resistance to the flow of blood secondary to constriction of small arteries throughout the body. Regulation of the level of blood pressure is dependent on a series of feed-back mechanisms in the largest artery, the aorta, and in the arteries to the brain. If pressures rise or fall above or below set levels, the degrees of constriction or dilation of the small aretries change automatically to maintain a given pressure, much as a thermostat regulates temperature. To a considerable extent, regulation of pressure is also under control of what is termed the sympathetic nervous system — accessory chains of nerves and nerve centres along the spinal column. These accessory nerves also help to regulate heart rate, certain hormonal functions, activity of the intestinal tract, and sweating.

In 1924 surgical removal of most of the sympathetic nervous system — sympathectomy — was initiated as a treatment for severe essential hypertension. At that time, there was no satisfactory effective medication to lower blood pressure, and an individual with the severe, rapidly progressive, so-called malignant form seldom lived more than a year after the presence of the disease was detected. It was known from animal experiments that stimulating sympathetic nerves increased vascular tone by causing constriction of small arteries, and that cutting these nerves caused them to dilate by relaxing vascular tone. The concept, supported by Walter Cannon, one of the outstanding physiologists of his time, was that overactivity of the sympathetic nervous system was a major factor in producing high blood pressure. After extensive surgical removal of the chains of nerve centres in the sympathetic nervous systems of dogs, there was an abrupt drop in blood pressure, but the pressure gradually returned to previous levels within a few weeks. With the observation that, in spastic paraplegic patients, the removal for other reasons of sympathetic nerve chains along the lower spine, the lumbar region, caused relaxation of vascular tone, Alfred Adson, a neurosurgeon at the Mayo Clinic, performed bilateral sympathectomy on a patient with severe high blood pressure in 1924. At first the pressure readings were much improved, though still above normal; the patient's headaches were relieved, and blurring of vision lessened so that he could read without difficulty. Six months later he was still in good health, but his severe elevation of blood pressure had returned.

This partial success led other surgeons to try this approach. The fact that relief of elevation of the pressure was temporary was thought to be due to inadequate resection of the sympathetic nerves; therefore, the operation was extended to include those along the ribs near the spine. During the thirties, a series of techniques was devised with varying success, all designed to cut permanently the sympathetic nerve supply to the small arteries of a large area of the body in order to decrease the total arterial resistance sufficiently to relieve the elevated pressure and thereby prolong life. In 1940 Adson reported 300 cases with no operative deaths. The results were disappointing in that, while symptoms were relieved, the good pressure responses obtained in those without "fixed" high pressure did not last for more than a few years. In the forties, many other surgeons in both the United States and Europe performed sympathectomies with variable results. A well-known surgeon at the Massachusetts General Hospital, Reginald Smithwick, became the chief advocate of the operation from 1938 through the 1940s. By 1953 he had operated on 2,400 patients, with an operative mortality of only 2.5 per cent, and was enthusiastic regarding his results; about 45 per cent of his surviving patients had significantly lowered blood pressure in the early years after surgery. Dr. Smithwick and his co-workers also made careful comparisons of patients treated medically and by sympathectomy, which indicated to them that the operation prolonged life. Similar results were reported from Sweden. Comparisons were made with unoperated patients who had refused surgery; but comparisons with concurrent controls treated at random were never made, and others have criticised the comparability of the patients who had undergone surgery and those who had not. Surgeons in England, operating only severe cases, reported discouraging results, concluding in effect that if the hypertension was mild, surgery was not necessary; and if severe, surgery did not work.

In 1960 a group of internists at the Massachusetts General Hospital did a meticulous, sophisticated statistical analysis of the results ten years after surgery in 100 consecutive patients operated by Smithwick and his associates. Lacking concurrent controls for comparisons, they selected records of patients with hypertension treated medically at the same period but at several institutions, matching them with the surgical records with respect to age; sex; degree of elevation of blood pressure; other findings from physical examination; laboratory data such as electrocardiogram, x-ray, and blood chemistry; and significant complications such as strokes. It was a retrospective study carried out with utmost care. Their conclusion was that 1 in 5 of the operated patients had lasting benefit, compared to 1 in 100 of the medically treated patients; that some dramatically favourable results occurred following surgery. But the effect on life expectancy was disappointing.

Forty-one per cent of the surgical patients had died, compared to forty-eight per cent of the medical patients. In view of the fact that the selection was not random and the treatment not strictly concurrent, it is impossible to know if this difference is significant. There is little doubt that the surgery was effective in a minority of patients, but it was impossible to predict in advance which ones they were. It is not clear even today whether the operation prolongs life.

A Pain Reliever for Arthritis

An illustration of the possibility of over-reaction is presented by the history of a useful drug which may have been abandoned on the basis of insufficient evidence.

Like phenacetin, cincophen is a synthetic chemical for reduction of fever and relief of pain, particularly useful for arthritis and gout. It was introduced in 1908 and quickly became popular and widely used as a prescription drug and as a constituent of many patent medicines, both on the North American continent and throughout Europe, employed much as aspirin and phenacetin are, for headaches, colds, neuralgia, toothaches, fevers, in addition to arthritis and gout. In 1932 one reviewer listed thirty-two combinations containing cincophen as the active ingredient; four years later the annual production in the United States totalled 90,000 pounds.

The first case of jaundice associated with the use of cincophen was reported in 1923. Thereafter, there was a gradual increase in the numbers of cases throughout the mid-thirties; then the numbers decreased, disappearing in the early forties. One reviewer stated in 1948 that 230 cases had been placed on record, 101 of which were fatal, death being due to severe liver disease of a type then called acute yellow atrophy. The assumption by most physicians then and now is that there is a cause and effect relationship, and for this reason, use of the drug has been virtually abandoned.

But the epidemiological facts do not indicate that a casual association was ever established, for the following reasons:

1. The existence of an epidemic was never clearly demonstrated. The disease did not differ on the basis of any then available diagnostic methods — laboratory, or post mortem — from the so-called catarrhal jaundice (now termed viral hepatitis). Then as now, the prevalence of viral hepatitis varied considerably from time to time and place to place, so that there was no base line to indicate that there had been an increase in the number of cases of jaundice beyond that expected in the population. Also, there was no significant change in the total number of deaths reported in the United States as being due to acute yellow atrophy, over a ten-year period. On the other hand, the high mortality rate was not typical of viral hepatitis.

2. The onset of jaundice was poorly related to the time of ingestion of the drug and amount taken. Some patients became ill within a few days of using cincophen; in others, jaundice did not appear for many months. Similarly, there was no relationship between the amount taken and the likelihood of developing the disease, unlike analgesic nephropathy associated with abuse of phenacetin. Small doses were sometimes followed by death, whereas large doses were often well tolerated for years.

3. Notwithstanding the fact that more cincophen was consumed in Europe than in the United States, most of the cases of jaundice were reported from the United States. In addition, on a year-to-year basis, the amount of the drug sold in thousands of pounds was not clearly related to the numbers of cases of liver disease.

4. Finally, two large series of cases of arthritis were reported, each with several thousand patients, in which there were no cases of jaundice, in spite of long-term treatment with the drug. In a comparison made on large numbers of arthritic

patients in one hospital between 1921 and 1935, there were ten cases of jaundice among those who had received cincophen against twenty among those who had not.

Experimentally in animals, it was not possible to reproduce the disease by administering cincophen, in spite of repeated attempts in several species — mice, rats, rabbits, dogs, and monkeys. (The drug does produce peptic ulcers in dogs.)

In 1941 the Council on Pharmacy and Chemistry of the American Medical Association concluded that the case against cincophen was not proven and suggested need for controlled clinical trials. None have been done; indeed, it is doubtful that it would be ethical to do so now. In 1964 two internists from the department of medicine at Harvard reviewed the problem, and in an editorial entitled "Drug or Viral," they agreed that the matter had never been settled.

It is quite possible that this useful but non-essential drug was given up prematurely and that the association between its use and the occurrence of jaundice was coincidental. Today, with better laboratory diagnostic tests and more sophisticated pathological studies, it might be possible to determine whether such jaundiced patients had viral or toxic hepatitis.

Anticoagulants in Coronary Heart Disease

Patients with arteriosclerosis of the coronary arteries which supply the heart muscle are susceptible to the pain of angina due to limitation of blood supply, or to heart attack with death of some portion of the heart muscle (myocardial infarction). For a quarter of a century in most countries, anticoagulant drugs to inhibit blood clotting have been used on patients with these problems; yet the value of this treatment is still debated. Some former enthusiasts have abandoned this treatment, believing that, overall, more harm than good has resulted. It is of interest to consider it as an example of the extremely difficult problem of evaluating some forms of treatment, and, in addition, it illustrates most of the problems relating to controlled clinical trials.

Experimental work on dogs in 1939 demonstrated that the

anticoagulant drug heparin, injected intravenously, could prevent the formation of clots occurring after the major branch of the left coronary artery was ligated. At that time, however, there was no drug which could be given by mouth; so it was not until 1945 that a practical clinical trial could be made of the new anticoagulants suitable for oral administration. The basic concept was that clotting played an important role as a major contributing factor increasing the obstructions in the coronary arteries, either after heart attacks, or in patients with angina pectoris. The assumption was made that life could be prolonged, and that blood clot formation in the hearts of these patients, producing further obstructions of the coronary arteries — as well as strokes and pulmonary emboli — could be prevented largely by keeping patients on anticoagulants for a period of months or years.

Encouraging initial results led in 1948 to a planned major controlled clinical trial involving 800 patients. The trial was carried out with the co-operation of the American Heart Association and sixteen hospitals, and careful statistical analyses were made. The control group was comprised of 368 patients; the treated group, 432. Patients were comparable with respect to age, sex, history of previous myocardial infarctions, and severity of present attacks (this last depended entirely on the clinical judgment of the physicians caring for the patients). Treatment was similar, except that the control patients did not receive antigoagulants. However, in spite of the fact that the influential English statistician, Bradford Hill, had carefully detailed the necessary components of a well-designed clinical trial ten years previously, several important principles were disregarded. Two deserve special mention. The method of insuring random allocation of patients to control and treatment groups consisted of treating the patients admitted to the co-operating hospitals on odd days with anticoagulants, and those admitted on even days with no anticoagulants. The referring and admitting physicians thus knew in advance which treatment their patient would receive, and by deferring admission appropriately, these doctors could choose for their patients the form of therapy which they believed more beneficial. The other basic deficiency of this important and influential study was that it was not double-blind. The physicians admitting, caring for, and evaluating the patient all knew not only who was to be treated, but who had been treated. The results indicated that the use of anticoagulants reduced the death rate, the number of new infarctions, and the incidence of complications resulting from thrombi such as strokes and pulmonary emboli. Bleeding — from the intestinal tract, into the lungs, around the heart — is a known hazard of the use of any drugs that retard the coagulation or clotting of the blood, yet only one serious hemorrhage occurred among the 432 treated patients.. Therefore, the authors concluded, "Anticoagulant therapy should be used in all cases of coronary thrombosis with myocardial infarction unless a definite contraindication exists."

This form of treatment, though widely adopted, caused intense debate in the 1950s and 1960s. Many outstanding physicians strongly believed that it was mandatory and life-saving, while others argued that complications outweighed possible advantages. Its use requires periodic supervision and careful regulation of medication, depending on the laboratory results of blood tests. Besides the expense and inconvenience, there is the ever-present risk of hemorrhage, which can be fatal. This disagreement led to forty-three large clinical trials during the following twenty-two years, involving thousands of patients. Some of these studies indicated that the treatment was advantageous, that life was prolonged, that complications related to clotting — such as strokes and pulmonary emboli — were less, and that the hazards of bleeding due to the drugs used were outweighed by the benefits. Other reports were inconclusive or indicated that the harm done outweighed the benefits. They illustrate the difficult problems inherent in the evaluation of the treatment, of a highly variable and unpredictable condition when the results are not dramatic.

Two investigators in the department of medicine at Yale, Robert Gifford and Alvan Feinstein, in 1969 made a critique of the methods used in thirty-two trials of the use of anticoagulants in acute myocardial infarction during the first weeks after the attack (the period when death is most common). They applied a series of standards now generally regarded as necessary for insuring that the patients in each group are comparable and that bias is minimized. These include:

1. *Standardization of diagnostic criteria.* There is no single diagnostic laboratory test of a myocardial infarction. The diagnosis rests on both clinical findings and laboratory tests including the electrocardiogram and several types of blood tests. Gifford and Feinstein pointed out that it is essential that the specific criteria for diagnosis be clearly established in advance and that they be the same for all physicians involved, so that one investigator could be replaced by another, if necessary. In most of these studies, only general guidelines were followed.

2. *Establishment of a plan in advance.* Three-fifths of the thirty-two studies were not planned. They were surveys comparing cases collected from routine medical records of patients treated according to the discretion of the individual attending physician.

3. *Concurrent controls.* This feature is considered to be one of the most important in a proper clinical trial — that patients in the treatment and control groups be cared for at the same time. Many changes in diagnosis and in ancillary medical care occur with the passage of time, so that better results, which have nothing to do with the specific therapy being evaluated, often are recorded in the later group, because of improved general care. Most physicians are unaware of these changes. Almost a quarter of the trials in various hospitals were not concurrent.

4. *Comparability of ancillary treatment.* It is obvious though often forgotten, that all care, other than the treatments being compared, should be identical. This is easy to accomplish when the trial is being carried on in one hospital or institution; but, when many institutions are involved, as is often the case, special efforts must be made in advance to insure comparability of treatment.

5. *Random allocation of patients to treatment groups.* This feature has already been discussed in connection with the early American Heart Association trial. In only four of the studies were the patients appropriately randomized to avoid bias.

6. *Appropriate division and comparison of sub-groups.* As nearly as possible, patients who are equally ill with initially similarly significant complications should be compared. The good-risk patients in one group should not be compared to the poor-risk patients in another. Only about half the reports satisfied this criterion.

7. *Use of double-blind approach.* It is true that in the use of anticoagulant drugs the doctor regulating the doses in accordance with laboratory findings must be aware of the patient's treatment. However, the doctors evaluating the results of the forms of treatment can remain unaware, "blind," objective. Only one of the thirty-two studies reviewed was carried out according to an appropriate double-blind procedure.

The results from the thirty-two studies revealed that fourteen concluded that anticoagulants were of value, and thirteen concluded that they were not. Using the criteria and standards listed above, Gifford and Feinstein found that the more closely the criteria were adhered to, the more likely the conclusion that anticoagulants were not advantageous.

Subsequently, in 1972 a group of cardiologists at the Albert Einstein College of Medicine in New York extended this approach to include long-term anticoagulant treatment carried on for months or years. Eleven studies were analyzed, all of which were planned in advance and used concurrent controls; however, they varied with respect to the other criteria, and no study fulfilled all of them. These authors concluded that a study could be planned and carried out to answer the important question of whether anticoagulants are truly beneficial in preventing heart attacks and their complications. The cardiologists added, however, that further studies were not warranted because of the following:

1. The long experience of previous studies has been largely inconclusive.

2. The present evidence is that the anticoagulant drugs used are effective only in preventing clotting in veins, and that they do not adequately inhibit clotting in arteries.

3. Recent data indicate that clots in the coronary arteries follow rather than cause acute myocardial infarction.

4. The present experience of coronary care confirms that, with regard to acute heart attacks, there appears to be a fixed mortality, not possible to lower by therapy.

In spite of this uncertainty and these arguments, most cardiologists continue to use anticoagulants, but in a limited fashion — some employing them only during the two- or three-week hospitalization of the patient, when the infarction has been severe, or in the presence of certain rhythm disturbances. Many continue to give them almost routinely for periods of two or three years, despite the fact that there is now little evidence to show that anticoagulants prevent coronary thrombosis and recurrent infarction. But the present trend is to restrict their use to selected cases, and few doctors agree completely as to exactly what the criteria of selection should be.

Is this form of treatment an error, in that the benefits gained do not outweigh the harm? Perhaps we shall never know. Nevertheless, as the authors of a leading text on cardiology, *The Heart,* wrote in 1970; "The 'anticoagulant era' seems to be coming to an end."

Evidence other than that derived from clinical trials appears to be causing the treatment to be given up.

A Drug to Prevent Migraine Headaches

Methysergide was a drug widely used for fifteen years which produced serious side effects and whose benefits in treatment of a disease were never carefully balanced against the harmful results. Migraine was the disease.

So typical are most attacks of this fascinating but unpleasant disease that it was clearly recognized as an entity in Greco-Roman times, 2,000 years ago — one of the oldest known illnesses. While its cause and cure remain unknown, symptomatic treatment is often effective in relieving the periodic painful, throbbing, one-sided headaches, which may be preceded by visual disturbances — spots or coloured lights — and followed by nausea and vomiting. The attacks may occur several times a week, or two or three times in a lifetime, the frequency of their occurrence often being influenced by psychological or emotional disturbances. Between attacks, patients are nearly always healthy and productive. (A disproportionate number of artists, scientists, and doctors appear to be afflicted.) Inasmuch as about one in twenty adults suffers from the disease, it is an important problem; those with the disabling headaches believe it is a highly important one. But the variability with respect to frequency and severity of migraine attacks, and the well-known effects of emotional and psychological disturbances make it extremely difficult to evaluate the efficacy of dugs for treatment or prevention. More than 400 remedies, including surgery, have been claimed to be helpful for this condition.

In 1894 William Thompson, a New York physician, learned by accident that the drug ergot, extracted from a fungus parasite of wheat, seemed to dramatically relieve attacks of "periodic neuralgia." The toxic effects of ergot have been known since the Middle Ages, when it was the cause of suffering and death. Bread contaminated by the fungus and eaten produced ergot poisoning, resulting in fiery redness and gangrene of the extremities, and sometimes loss of limb and life — the disease called St. Anthony's fire. The present theory is that migraine headaches are due to dilation of the arteries in the head. Non-toxic amounts of ergot compounds are thought to constrict these arteries. The drug ergotamine came into general use for migraine in 1928. It is the only drug usually effective in managing a severe attack, but even response to it is not consistently greater than to a placebo in planned controlled trials. Also, it must be given promptly at the onset of an attack. Toxic reactions to it do occur, and the use of ergotamine is avoided in most types of blood-vessel disease such as hypertension and coronary arteriosclerosis. Some persons are highly sensitive to it.

For many years the hope was of finding a method of preventing migraine attacks. In 1959 a synthetic compound, methysergide, related in its molecular structure to both ergot and lysergic acid (LSD), was introduced, and appeared to have unquestionable value in preventing or greatly reducing the frequency of headaches in upwards of 90 per cent of the patients who could tolerate the drug. However, as Oliver Sachs, a neurologist at the Albert Einstein College of Medicine in New York, commented in his monograph on migraine: "It was widely held that the wonder drug for migraine had at last arrived; the expectation of its healing powers doubtless contributed to those powers. However, its efficacy and its reputation have both declined over the years; in unison, it may now be said that methysergide benefits no more than a third of all patients with frequent severe migraines."

Within a few years after its introduction, methysergide became widely used; an estimated one million patients received it. In 1964 John Graham, an internist at Harvard Medical School, observed what appeared to be a unique side effect of the chronic administration of methysergide — the development of a peculiar fibrous, scarlike tissue change. Most often this fibrosis occurred in the tissue around the ureters, the tubes connecting the kidney with the bladder. Constriction of these tubes produced partial obstruction to the flow of urine and impaired kidney function. Following publication of the initial report, a series of articles appeared confirming the association of this condition with chronic administration of methysergide, and indicating that fibrosis with scarring and thickening of tissue could also occur in the lungs, on heart valves, and in large arteries, producing partial obstruction. The existence of a causal relationship between the drug and the fibrosis was confirmed by the fact that the manifestations — pains, urinary obstruction, heart murmurs — nearly always disappeared spontaneously when the drug was discontinued. On the few occasions when it was restarted the signs and symptoms recurred. Also, there seemed to be a direct relationship with the duration of treatment, no case occuring less than four months after starting it. By 1969 there had been about 200 reports of this toxic reaction. It was estimated that this side effect occurred in about 1 one per cent of the patients taking methysergide for prolonged periods. While most persons suffering from these complications completely recovered, many experienced weeks or months of pain and discomfort. Some required abdominal surgery; one had a heart valve replaced.

In 1973 the advice on methysergide was to limit the use of the drug to patients handicapped by frequent severe attacks which fail to respond to other drugs; to give it no longer than six months continuously; and to perform physical examinations, electrocardiograms, and x-ray studies of the kidneys, ureters, and bladder. The assumption is that the benefits of the drug outweigh the hazards in these cases.

What is now surprising is the fact that methysergide's efficacy in this variable disease was never adequately tested. Double-blind and single-blind studies have been carried out on a small scale, with variable results. Clinical trials without controls have been made with many patients. But there has not been an adequate, carefully planned controlled clinical trial, with random allocation of patients to placebo and treatment groups, to really test the effectiveness of methysergide in the prevention of migraine headaches.

CHAPTER SIX

Lessons

The mistakes presented in this account have produced impressive and dramatic changes in testing, in recognition, in legislation, in scientific knowledge, and in public attitudes as well as the attitudes of doctors and scientists. For the most part, these changes have occurred since the 1930s. Only a few *new* lessons have been learned; by and large, the errors have served in a tragic fashion to remind men of known truths and to emphasize those truths.

Need for Testing: Value of Animal Trials

Once a remedy or treatment has been devised or proposed, after due consideration of the pertinent information and the basic laboratory data — chemical, biochemical, biophysical, physiological — the next step is to test the treatment under consideration on animals in order to determine its feasibility, effectiveness, and range of dose, as well as its toxicity. While safety is a prime consideration, a determination must be made as to whether the treatment — surgical or medical — is practical and will produce the desired results. Primitive man undoubtedly tested food, drugs, and poisons on animals before trying them himself, but careful scientific animal trials to evaluate treatment began early in the 19th century by François Magendie, a brilliant neurophysiologist and pharmacologist. He recognized the basic similarity of living organisms, but, while he tested many substances for their toxic and physiologic effects, believing that "the manner of action of medicines and poisons is the same on man as on animals," he made no effort to evaluate the curative values of drugs. The most famous of the early systematic tests were those carefully done by Louis Pasteur to test the efficacy of his vaccine for the prevention of anthrax in 1881. Sixty sheep were used; twenty-five were inoculated with the vaccine and then infected, twenty-five were infected only, and ten were neither inoculated nor infected. All the uninoculated and infected died, and all the inoculated survived. Such conclusive results are rarely obtained.

In the 20th century the use of extensive, careful trials, both controlled and uncontrolled, on a wide variety of species of animals, has become accepted as an essential preliminary for screening medical and surgical treatments before employing them on man.

The examples presented here offered many illustrations of the use, misuse, and lack of use of animals for testing. Among the errors of concept Sir Almoth Wright's failures to make appropriate animal trials allowed valueless autogenous vaccines to be used for more than three decades. Erroneous conclusions drawn from poorly planned experiments by the bacteriologist Edward Rosenow were largely responsible for many of the follies resulting from the theory of focal infection.

The same was true for the surgeons who revascularized hearts and brains, froze stomachs, and glued fractures. All of them worked with animals, testing their concepts and their techniques on animals before operating on patients. Yet, as we have seen, after hundreds of persons had been treated or operated on, more critical experiments and trials on animals by other investigators helped substantially to disprove the effectiveness and value of their procedures.

Three painfully obvious demonstrations of the need and value of testing drugs for toxicity were the catastrophes resulting from the use of "elixir of sufanilamide," stalinon, and triparanol (MER 29). In the first two of these, relatively simple animal tests performed after the tragedies made obvious the highly toxic nature of the industrial solvent diethylene glycol, and the tin compound, di-ethyl tin di-iodide. The toxicity of the third — its tendency to produce cataracts — was known before it was released for administration to patients, but the information was withheld.

Thalidomide, as we have seen, is a special problem. There is little question that its toxicity could have been detected by appropriate animal trials. Deformities similar to phocomelia had been produced in both monkeys and in one strain of rabbits by giving the drug to pregnant females of those species. Indeed, the necessity for testing of drugs for teratogenicity was one of the important lessons resulting from the tragedy. But such a need was not generally recognized before it happened, and it was not common practice to test in this fashion at that time. Another lesson learned was the advisability of testing for ill effects of long-term (six months to a year or more) chronic administration of a drug to animals, if it is to be given to patients for similar periods. It is likely that the polyneuritis, the other serious side effect of thalidomide, could have been anticipated and avoided, had chronic tests been done. Again, such trials were not the usual practice at the time, though psychotropic drugs were often tested in this way. The *acute* toxicity of thalidomide had been tested in mice, rats, dogs, and monkeys before the drug was used on man.

The disasters resulting from overdose and abuse of drugs demonstrated other aspects of the value of animal testing. If medication is going to be used in larger than conventional doses, or for longer than usual periods of time, it should be tested accordingly. Information from early experiments on rats should have warned clinicians of the possible dangers of the long-continued large amounts of vitamin D given to patients with arthritis and tuberculosis. The production of a disease similar to SMON in dogs given large amounts of clioquinol for a long period of time indicates that the catastrophic epidemic of that disease in Japan might have been prevented had such testing been done before the doctors and public abused the drug by administering it for months. A special lesson was that derived from the blindness produced by exposing premature infants to high concentrations of oxygen. The experimental production of similar blindness in newborn kittens by exposure to oxygen in the same way not only furnished evidence of the cause of retrolental fibroplasia, it dramatically emphasized the need to test treatment specifically in animals of the same biological age that will be applied in patients, particularly in the premature and the newborn — a need previously ignored.

Another special example was the evidence gained from giving dogs isoproteronol after the concentration in their arterial oxygen saturation had been lowered to mimic the effects of an asthmatic attack. The resulting slowing of the heart and cardiac arrest offered a plausible explanation of the sudden deaths associated with the use of aerosol inhalants.

To a high degree clinical tests forecast reliably most of the serious side effects of drugs. Often they allow the investigator to know if the drug will be effective. An overall analysis was made of their predictive value in Switzerland between 1959 and 1962. Of 100 new drugs of varying types, clinical trial confirmed the efficacy and toxicity anticipated from the animal studies in 75 per cent. However, essential and valuable as animal trials are, they have limitations even when carried out with the searching sophisticated techniques used today.

Some of the limitations of animal trials are:

Species differences. More than a thousand years ago, Avicenna, the renowned Persian physician who compiled the influential *Canon,* the great medical textbook of its time, wrote, "The test must be done on the human body, for trying a drug on a lion or a horse might not prove anything about its effect on man." Several examples of side effects are discussed here. In repeated attempts, investigators were unsuccessful in trying to cause acrodynia by the use of calomel in teething powders, cataracts with dinitrophenol, permanent pulmonary hypertension with aminorex, nephropathy with phenacetin. Thousands of animals, including rats, mice, and monkeys, failed to develop the viral hepatitis produced by certain lots of yellow fever vaccine, since the virus is specific for Man.

It is often impossible to duplicate in animals the disease or condition to be treated in Man. This is one of the commonest problems. It is quite feasible to reproduce in animals most of the bacterial infectious diseases common to Man — streptococcal infections, tuberculosis, yellow fever, staphylococcal infections — in one species or another of the laboratory animals commonly used. Vitamin deficiencies — rickets, scurvy, pellagra, etc. — can be caused and treated. In recent years much ingenuity has gone into efforts to duplicate in animals conditions or diseases that are chiefly human. Many forms of cancer, a type of arthritis, atherosclerosis, peptic ulcer, and certain behaviour patterns can be produced in animals, then studied and treated. But conditions such as rheumatoid arthritis, mental retardation, bronchial asthma, many of the mental illnesses, essential hypertension, coronary atherosclerosis (as it appears in man) or migraine cannot be successfully mimicked.

In the past decade, testing of drugs on animals has become far more sophisticated than in previous times, radically increasing the value of this approach. Drugs which are excreted from the body unchanged — usually chemicals which are not fat soluble — with few exceptions affect man and other mammals in the same fashion. On the other hand, substances which break down and undergo bio-transformation often affect different species, even different individuals of the same species, in a highly variable fashion. The differences result largely from the metabolic handling of the drug in the body — the way in which it is absorbed, broken down and excreted — rather than from its physiological effects on tissues which are remarkably similar among mammalian species. When the effects of drugs are related to their levels in the blood or tissues, most of the apparent variations disappear. By determining these levels, the value and reliability of animal testing are greatly enhanced. Further support is given by tracing the breakdown of chemicals and the deposition in various organs of the body, employing radioactive tagged isotopes. The use of several animal species also helps to avoid the false conclusion either that a remedy will be too toxic to Man, or that it will be ineffective. One classic example is that of penicillin, which is highly toxic to guinea pigs in small doses, but which can be given in very large amounts safely to man and other animals.

Teratogenic effects of drugs vary widely from one species to another. For example, aspirin in large doses readily produces deformities of the fetus in rats, but has not been known to do so in Man. In this respect, as well as in many others involving both toxicity and efficacy, animal trials may be misleading and may prevent an important beneficial treatment from being tried on Man. It is impossible to know what we may be missing by setting up restrictive animal trials as a hurdle. However, at present all known teratogenic agents, physical and chemical, affecting Man, also affect commonly used laboratory animals, if equivalent doses are used. Further, many differences between Man and other mammals will disappear if conditions are made comparable for the conditions to be treated; that is, if the tests on animals are made with doses substantially less than those known to be toxic, and if the drugs are used in a similar fashion as they would be in Man.

The communication barrier. The inability of animals to talk is an obstacle which prevents proper evaluation of responses involving pain, discomfort, subjective sensations, decision making, memory, and all but the lower aspects of the intellect. It is particularly difficult to test the efficacy of sedatives such as thalidomide, analgesics such as phenacetin, and certain surgical procedures designed to increase mental acuity, such as revascularization of the brain.

Idiosyncratic toxicity. This is usually difficult and often impossible to detect either by animal trials or by trials made on human beings. If a reaction occurs but once in every hundred individuals, several hundred subjects will be required in both the treated and the control groups to discover the difference. If it occurs once in a thousand, several thousand subjects will be needed. Further, since the tests must be duplicated whenever a new species or dose of drug is introduced, it is not practical to use the tests except for measuring reactions present in more than 5 per cent of the animals. Perhaps this phenomenon of idiosyncracy even more than species differences may account for the inability of investigators to duplicate acrodynia, dinitrophenol cataracts, pulmonary hypertension, hypercalcemia (except with very high doses of vitamin D), and analgesic nephropathy.

Long-delayed reactions. This problem has been clearly recognized only in the past few years. When the possibility of delayed reaction is suspected, animals are observed for six months to a year after the administration of a drug is stopped. Also, careful autopsy examination of all the important organs with special microscopic studies is made in the attempt to detect hidden damage. Nevertheless, certain severe toxic effects analyzed here could hardly have been predicted. They include cancer of the thyroid gland which developed in the children who had been irradiated as infants and which did not appear until many years later, and cancer of the vagina in the daughters of mothers given stilbestrol during pregnancy and which did not appear until the daughters were in their teens.

Erect posture. With the exception of the higher primates, man is alone in walking erect. This is seldom a consideration, but this unique feature did prevent the theories of visceroptosis and its treatments from being tested on the usual laboratory animals.

After sufficient data concerning a method of treatment — probable efficacy, feasibility, dose range, toxic reactions — have been obtained, the next step is a preliminary trial in human beings. This may be cautiously performed on a few healthy volunteers, or on patients with the disease to be treated. It must depend on the situation. Last and most important, whenever possible, before treatments are applied to the public at large, should come the planned controlled clinical trials.

Need for Testing: Value of Controlled Clinical Trials on Patients

This most useful of all tools for testing the efficacy as well as the ill effects of most new treatments should precede their general use. In its present form, the technique constitutes the major advance in the science of therapy. Much of the credit for its present use is due to a brilliant, persuasive Englishman, Sir Austin Bradford Hill, Fellow of the Royal Society and Professor of Medical Statistics at the University of London. Although not a physician, Hill has done more than any individual to convince the medical profession that these tests are essential.

Clinical trials are as old as medicine itself, since observations of the effects of new treatments of patients were made by the earliest physicians. Much was gained in the past by keen observations on the part of astute observers noting carefully what happened after a change in therapy, comparing the new results with those occurring before the change. The original observations and cautious deductions recorded in the Hippocratic books were outstanding achievements, the use of morphine, mercurials, quinine, and digitalis resulted from observation and deduction; comparisons of changes in individual patients were made following therapy and after its discontinuance. Theories based on contemporary knowledge of physics and chemistry, biology, and physiology guided and often misguided treatment. Equally often, the clinical experience of the eminent physician or professor determined what was used or how surgery was performed.

In spite of the explosion of scientific thought and experiment in Europe in the 1500s and 1600s, a simple, well-planned, con-

139

trolled trial does not appear to have taken place until 1747, when John Lind, a Scottish naval surgeon, made a classic comparative trial of the current "cures" for scurvy. As many as three-quarters of the men on long voyages died of this dread disease. Lind describes it briefly, in his classic, *A Treatise of the Scurvy*: "On the 20th of *May,* 1747, I took twelve patients in the scurvy, on board the *Salisbury* at sea. Their cases were as similar as I could have them. They all in general had putrid gums, the spots and lassitude, with weakness of their knees. They lay together in one place, being a proper apartment for the sick in the fore-hold; and had one diet common to all, *viz.* water-gruel sweetened with sugar in the morning; fresh mutton-broth often times for dinner; at other times puddings, boiled biscuits with sugar, etc. And for supper, barley and raisins, rice and currants, sago and wine, or the like. Two of these were ordered each a quart of cyder a day. Two others took twenty-five gutts of *elixir vitriol* three times a day, upon an empty stomach; using a gargle strongly acidulated with it for their mouths. Two others took two spoonfuls of vinegar three times a day, upon an empty stomach; having their gruels and their other food well acidulated with it, as also the gargle for their mouths. Two of the worst patients, with the tendons in the ham rigid (a symptom none of the rest had) were put under a course of sea-water. Of this they drank half a pint every day, and sometimes more or less as it operated, by way of gentle physic. Two others had each two oranges and one lemon given them every day. These they eat with greediness, at different times, upon an empty stomach. They continued but six days under this course, having consumed the quantity that could be spared. The two remaining patients, took the bigness of a nutmeg three times a day of an electuary recommended by a hospital- surgeon, made of garlic, mustard-feed, *rad. raphan,* balsam of *Peru,* and gum myrrh; using for common drink barley-water well acidulated with tamarinds; by a decoction of which, with the addition of *cremor tartar,* they were greatly purged three or four times during the course.

"The consequence was, that the most sudden and visible good effects were perceived from the use of the oranges and lemons; one of those who had taken them, being at the end of six days fit for duty. The spots were not indeed at that time quite off his body, nor his gums sound; but without an other medicine, than a gargle of *elixir vitriol,* he became quite healthy before we came into Plymouth, which was on the 16th June. The other was the best recovered of any in his condition; and being now deemed pretty well, was appointed nurse to the rest of the sick."

Notwithstanding these results, lemon and lime juice (hence the term "Limey") were not supplied to the British Navy until forty years later, when the Lords of the Admiralty were finally convinced by Lind's work.

The next well-considered approach, using numbers and making careful comparisons, was that of Pierre-Charles-Alexander Louis, the chief of the famous hospital, Hôtel Dieu, in Paris, and one of the great clinical teachers of his time. Bleeding, along with purging, had for centuries been standard treatment for many diseases. In 1835 Louis studied the effects of bloodletting upon seventy-eight cases of pneumonia, thirty-three cases of erysipelas, and twenty-three cases of inflammation of the throat. He found no appreciable differences in mortality or in duration of disease between patients bled and not bled, nor between those bled at different stages of the diseases. This result was so contrary to orthodox teaching of the time that it caused an uproar among his colleagues in Paris. Even Louis was reluctant to accept his own results and continued to treat certain diseases with bloodletting. Nevertheless, his observation led to a decreased use of this unhappy form of therapy.

Louis' comments on his "Numerical Method" in the assessment of treatment are pertinent: "As to different methods of treatment, if it is possible for us to assure ourselves of the superiority of one or other among them in any disease whatever, having regard to the different circumstances of age, sex, and temperament, of strength and weakness, it is doubtless to be done by enquiring if under these circumstances a greater number of individuals have been cured by one means than another. Here again it is necessary to count. And it is, in great part at least, because hitherto this method has been not at all, or rarely employed, that the science of therapeutics is still so uncertain; that when the application of the means placed in our hands is useful we do not know the bounds of this utility . . . in order that the calculation may lead to useful or true results it is not sufficient to take account of the modifying powers of the individual; it is also necessary to know with precision at what period of the disease the treatment has been commenced; and especially we ought to know the natural progress of the disease, in all its degrees, when it is abandoned to itself, and whether the subjects have or have not committed errors of regimen; with other particulars."

Shyrock, the American medical historian, has pointed out that this constituted the introduction of mathematical procedures into clinical medicine, and called it the "most significant study ever made in the medical method."

About ten years later, an American physician, Elisha Bartlett, an admirer of Louis, formulated most of the basic principles of the modern controlled trial, stating that: "In therapeutic investigations cases which are to be compared must have equal disturbing factors of location, social class, and the like; they should be susceptible of a clear and positive diagnosis; there must be no selection of cases; and the method of treatment must be clearly defined. The certainty of results will be in proportion to the fixed and uniform character of the compared facts and to the greatness of their numbers. . . . No acquaintance, however perfect, with laws of pathology and therapeutics, can ever remove, or in any degree diminish, the necessity of a thorough and discriminating study and knowledge of the single instances which unite to make up the materials of the law."

During the rest of the 19th century, a number of physicians and surgeons, including the great surgeon Lister, used Louis' methods of counting and meticulous observation, but comparisons were nearly always made with a series of patients cared for prior to the new method of treatment. This approach is effective only when the differences are great, or when applied to highly fatal diseases such as meningitis or diabetes. No concurrent controls were required to prove the effectiveness of penicillin or insulin in these diseases.

With the introduction of antisera and vaccines, many trials were made comparing control and treated groups observed simultaneously. Nearly all of these failed to fulfill modern criteria for well-planned tests; the numbers of cases were frequently too small; patients in the control and treated groups were frequently not matched with respect to age, symptoms, or severity; assignment of patients to each group was frequently not done in a random fashion;

observations or results were seldom made in a uniform way because many observers were involved. Calmette's trials of BCG were examples of these errors. Nevertheless, because the results were often dramatic, much progress was made in the prevention and treatment of infections. Often correct conclusions were arrived at for the wrong reasons, however, there were in addition many inconclusive results due to poor planning. The refusal of Sir Almoth Wright to test his clinical results by statistical analysis led to four decades of worthless vaccine therapy.

In the 1920s, two large-scale trials were carried out in a single-blind fashion to test immunization against the common cold. The effects of injection of the vaccine were compared with those of saline used as a placebo in two equal groups of volunteer students chosen at random. The students were blind in the respect that only the research worker knew which had received the saline and which the vaccine injections. This employment of a placebo on a large scale was a new step. The students in the treated group proved to be as susceptible to the colds as were the controls. About the same time, large-scale tests on patients with pneumonia demonstrated the effectiveness of the newly developed antisera.

According to J. B. Bull, who has traced their history, more clinical therapeutic trials have probably occurred since 1935 than in all previous time. That year Domagk introduced sulfanilamide in the form of Prontosil, and effective treatment of bacterial infections began. The need for testing was greater than ever before. Two years later Bradford Hill published the first edition of *Medical Statistics,* which clearly defined the principles and requirements of well-designed controlled clinical trials. This book, now in its tenth edition, together with his other writings and addresses, has been a major influence in the acceptance and refinement of this essential tool, which has both prevented and aborted many blunders of medical treatment, and in addition has clearly designated many effective methods.

Why were well-planned controlled clinical trials so long delayed? Avicenna, in the 9th century, had pointed out the need for comparison of similar groups of patients treated by different methods.

Bull, in his historical account, suggests three major reasons for the delay:

1. reverence for authority and tradition
2. lack of effective remedies.
3. the relationship of doctor and patient.

The first of these, reverence for authority and tradition, was a powerful deterrent to any form of testing for centuries. Deductions were made from premises made by Hippocrates and Galen, and enunciated by the professors in the universities. Methods of treatment were copied and translated from one text to another. To maintain the myth of infallibility, it was necessary to deny doubt and ignorance; the admission of doubt and ignorance is essential in order to recognize the need for controlled trials and to confirm that experience is often only perpetuation of error. The physician must acknowledge that he does not know if a new form of treatment is better than the old, or if an old one is good. He must be willing to be proven wrong.

The second of these reasons, the lack of effective remedies, greatly reduced the incentive to test drugs and methods. It is always more gratifying to show that something new works than to disprove an old established method. The developments in the 19th century in organic chemistry, biochemistry, and in bacteriology led to the development in the 20th century of a host of new products requiring critical evaluation. Also, the diagnostic tools which made such evaluations precise became available.

The last reason, the relationship of the doctor and patient is particularly responsible for the delay. This relationship continues to postpone the acceptance of critical evaluation and influences many physicians and most of the public. The relationship involves ethical and moral considerations which require special discussion. It is natural and proper for the doctor to feel that he must treat the individual patient in the best way, without interference. The patient needs to have confidence that this is the case. Both must feel that everything is being done with whatever means are available, and that it is unethical to withhold a treatment which may be of benefit. Consequently, there is again a reluctance to admit doubt and ignorance, to realize that what is new is not always best, and to recognize that each treatment is a trial involving uncertainties of hazards as well as benefits. There is the additional reluctance on the part of the doctor to surrender some of his authority for care of his patient, for large, planned controlled clinical trials involve many doctors and must offer a pre-set plan. Even in small trials limited to a single institution it is often necessary to have one set of physicians supervise and administer treatment, and another set, unaware of the particular treatment given, evaluate the results in order to achieve a double blind. Most of the objections can be overcome if guidelines are carefully observed.

Consent to participate in a trial must be freely given by the patient, after careful and fair explanation of its nature, together with possible benefits and hazards. It must involve understanding as well as willingness. The exceptions apply to children in instances in which there is a need to test a vaccine developed primarily for children, as in the case of poliomyelitis or tuberculosis, and to some patients in mental institutions* when the effects of pschotropic drugs, neurosurgery, or forms of shock therapy are to be tested. In those instances, the consent of parents or relatives must be obtained. It is also prudent and of practical value to have the agreement of the referring physician.

The trial should be carried out only when the information to be gained justifies the effort, after due consideration of possible risks and benefits. It must be a treatment which, although its results remain in doubt after careful animal experiments, shows promise after a few initial uncontrolled tests on patients, but whose ultimate value — weighing the risks against possible benefits — is questionable.

The ethics of clinical trials have been given much consideration and thought. The statement of Immanuel Kant in his *Categorical Imperative* has been proposed as a guide: "Every man is to be respected as an absolute end in himself; and it is a crime against the dignity that belongs to him as a human being, to use him as a mere means for some external purpose." The patient must not be exploited.

Spodick, an American cardiologist, has reversed the objections of Sir Almoth Wright and many others, by stating, "I submit that it is unethical and, worse, immoral to use any new form of therapy

*Whenever possible, these patients should give their own consent.

without giving the patient a fifty-fifty chance of not getting it; that anything less than this may enthrone Error; that anything less must be rejected, in fact scorned."

All aspects of medical care for the treatment group and the control groups must be the same and the best available, except for the method or medication being tested. The safety and well-being of the patient must always be the chief consideration, and the trial should be modified or abandoned if the form of therapy clearly proves either unduly hazardous or overwhelmingly beneficial.

Objective, disinterested, and impartial guidance must be employed in the planning, conduct, and interpretation of the results of the trial. The enthusiastic investigator who originates a new operation, procedure, or drug, cannot be a proper judge of his enterprise. Nor can the drug company which anticipates a profit if the results are favourable.

The comments of Henry Beecher, Professor of Research in anaesthesia and a critic of medical ethics, regarding the use of a double-blind trial in disproving the value of producing a new blood supply to the heart by ligation of the internal mammary arteries, illustrates this very well:

Some responsible physicians with the highest motives have said *they* could never carry out a sham procedure in any of *their* patients. Of course this can be done only with the full consent of the individuals involved, who must express a willingness not to know whether or not they were subjected to the full procedure until after the study is completed. The position of the high-minded physician or surgeon who says that he could never be a party to such a "sham procedure," however, is worthy of close consideration. He introduces a new treatment or operation — the subjective effects are particularly important here — which he and his colleagues and followers subsequently carry out hundreds of times. As with most major undertakings, some risk is involved: major surgery is always associated with a death rate. Then an equally high-minded investigator comes along who, *with the consent of his patients,* carries out a properly designed study which might in many cases consist of no more than twenty-five sham operations and twenty-five full procedures, for a total of fifty individuals. This investigator finds that the new procedure has no more power than a placebo, and its effects are transient at best. What then is the position of the high-minded physician or surgeon who refused to make such a clear-headed study? Those who have been subjected to his new procedure have lost a great deal of money and time. They have experienced discomfort and suffering, and several are dead. How, then, is the high-minded practitioner to face up to his failure to carry out a properly designed study? It does indeed seem at times that we are more considerate of our laboratory animals and their welfare than we are of the welfare and lives of our patients when we deny them an adequate test, when we subject them to the continuing risks of inadequately designed major therapeutic procedures.

The ethics of clinical trials and the principle of not exploiting human beings in order to gain scientific knowledge had been given careful consideration by physicians in the 19th century — particularly by Claude Bernard, the great French physiologist. But not until after the Second World War were formal codes of principles enunciated. The barbarous, inhumane, unproductive experiments carried out by the Nazis on human subjects caused much soul searching by men in both the medical and legal professions, for qualified German doctors had been involved in the Nazi atrocities. The Nuremberg Code in 1947 and the Declaration of Helsinki by the World Medical Association in 1964 were international efforts to formulate safeguards and standards to insure that the welfare of the patient is always the first consideration, and that wherever feasible, the consent of the patient be obtained.

Because some doctors and much of the public still fail to understand and continue to object to planned, controlled clinical trials, it is worth quoting part of a statement from the British Medical Research Council on the subject in 1962, "Control Subjects in Investigations of Treatment or Prevention":

> Over recent years, the development of treatment and prevention has been greatly advanced by the method of the controlled clinical trial. Instead of waiting, as in the past, on the

slow accumulation of general experience to determine the relative advantages and disadvantages of any particular measure, it is now often possible to put the question to the test under conditions which will not only yield a speedy and more precise answer, but also limit the risk of untoward effects remaining undetected. Such trials are, however, only feasible when it is possible to compare suitable groups of patients and only permissible when there is a genuine doubt within the profession as to which of two treatments or preventive regimes is the better. In these circumstances it is justifiable to give to a proportion of the patients the novel procedure on the understanding that the remainder receive the procedure previously accepted as the best. In the case when no effective treatment has previously been devised then the situation should be fully explained to the participants and their true consent obtained.

Such controlled trials may raise ethical points which may be of some difficulty. In general, the patients participating in them should be told frankly that two different procedures are being assessed and their cooperation invited. Occasionally, however, to do so is contra-indicated. For example, to awaken patients with a possibly fatal illness to the existence of such doubts about effective treatment may not always be in their best interest; or suspicion may have arisen as to whether a particular treatment has any effect apart from suggestion and it may be necessary to introduce a placebo into part of the trials to determine this. Because of these and similar difficulties, it is the firm opinion of the Council that controlled clinical trials should always be planned and supervised by a group of investigators and never by an individual alone. It goes without question that any doctor taking part in such a collective controlled trial is under an obligation to withdraw a patient from the trial, and to institute any treatment he considers necessary, should this, in his personal opinion, be in the better interests of his patient.

In the United States, when a new drug is involved, the FDA requires consent of the subject "except where the investigators deem it not feasible, or, in their professional judgement, contrary to the best interest of such human beings." The Helsinki Declaration and the Nuremberg Code are used as guidelines. The statement of the Helsinki Code is,

> If at all possible, consistent with patient psychology, the doctor should obtain the patient's freely given consent after the patient has been given a full explanation. In case of legal incapacity, consent should also be procured from the legal guardian; in case of physical incapacity the permission of the legal guardian replaces that of the patient.
>
> The doctor can combine clinical research with professional care, the objective being the acquisition of new medical knowledge, only to the extent that clinical research is justified by its therapeutic value for the patient.

Franz Ingelfinger, the editor of the influential *New England Journal of Medicine,* in a careful critical discussion of informed consent has pointed out that the patient seldom fully comprehends the precise nature and hazard of the clinical trial involved, but he argues that such consent does avoid the deceptions of the past. With keen perception he adds, "The subject's only real protection, the public as well as the medical profession must recognize, depends on the conscience and compassion of the investigator and his peers."

What of the other errors considered here? How many could have been avoided by the use of this tool? It seems probable that most of the errors of treatment resulting from the concepts of autointoxication and focal infection could have been demonstrated and would have limited the perpetuation of these mistakes. Hill, commenting on a problem still with us which relates to surgery, questioned, "Is it ethical to take the tonsils out of thousands of school children on the flimsiest of evidence and so unethical to conduct a controlled trial of the procedure to learn whether it has any value?" Vaccine therapy in rheumatoid arthritis was tested appropriately, but only after three decades of use. As has been recounted, this trial failed to indicate the superiority of the vaccine to the salt-water placebo.

It is likely that random allocation of infants with large thymuses and mild to moderate respiratory distress to equal control groups, and to groups treated by x-ray, would have shown lack of benefit, even though it would not have shown the rare cancers of the thyroid until more than ten years later. It even seems that the unfortunate results of the surgical attempt to revascularize the brain could have been limited to a small number of retarded children, rather than several hundred, had concurrent comparisons been made with similar patients not subjected to surgery. We have already seen how the ineffectiveness of freezing the stomach in the attempt to cure duodenal ulcer was exposed by a well-conducted double-blind controlled trial.

What of the catastrophes which resulted from the side effects of the drugs? The numbers of children poisoned as a result of the use of thallium paste for ringworm of the scalp could have been decreased, had this form of treatment been appropriately compared with the less convenient but well-accepted x-ray therapy. The early trials of dinitrophenol in the treatment of obesity included no concurrent controls. A limited planned trial with contemporary techniques and appropriate comparisons almost surely would have detected some of the serious toxic reactions as well as the ineffectiveness of dinitrophenol in weight reduction.

There is a real problem with respect to thalidomide. A careful well-planned short-term controlled trial comparing its effects as a sedative with those of barbiturates was conducted at the Johns Hopkins Hospital by one of the most reputable of the American clinical pharmacologists, Louis Lasagna. Given for a period of a few days to induce sleep, it was neither more nor less effective than barbiturates, with about as many side effects, none of which was severe. An English investigation arrived at similar conclusions. Many other clinical trials were performed, but these were nearly all poorly planned and uncontrolled, often sponsored by the drug company and little better than testimonials. In retrospect, it is apparent that since thalidomide was to be used on a long-term chronic basis in mental institutions, its effects should have been compared with those of one of the established drugs then in use, after administration over a period of many months. It is likely that its tendency to produce polyneuritis in some patients could have been demonstrated in this fashion. However, it must be admitted that in the late 1950s, most such sedatives were not tested in this manner, and drugs in general were not tested on pregnant female animals to determine if they affected the offspring.

The retrolental fibroplasia which blinded premature infants following their exposure to high concentrations of oxygen clearly could have been minimized by a very limited controlled clinical trial carried out early. This was made apparent by such tests made by Patz and his colleagues ten years after the epidemic began. The problem was that the clinicians failed to suspect that the premature infant might react differently. Beecher relates how this particular clinical trial illustrates some of the emotional reactions which frequently occur as a result of these tests. At the beginning, a number of the medical personnel involved were quite upset over the fact that the premature babies in the control group were being denied what were assumed to be the life-saving benefits of the high concentrations of oxygen. However, toward the end, when it began to appear that blindness occurred only to those exposed to oxygen, the same doctors and nurses were distressed about administering it to those being treated.

On the other hand, valuable as the clinical trial is, it has important limitations; chiefly the sometimes almost insurmountable difficulty of detecting reliably small but often highly important differences in effects on two treatment groups, and the difficulty in discovering the adverse effects which occur rarely. Uncertainties resulting from the attemps to evaluate the long-term use of anticoagulants illustrate the first of these limitations. Side effects resulting from idiosyncrasies or hypersensitivity occurring once in 500 cases or less illustrate the second, in such reactions as acrodynia, primary pulmonary hypertension, hypercalcemia, SMON, and phenacetin kidney damage. A third problem, much less common, is that it may be ethically impossible to conduct a planned controlled trial. Such would not have been possible with the use of different aerosol inhalants in varying doses for bronchial asthma when sudden death was suspected of being a hazard.

The next step in protection of patients from hazards and ill effects of therapy is the early recognition of these effects in order that suffering can be minimized and mistakes corrected.

151

Recognition and Monitoring — the Role of Epidemiology

Even the best clinical trials involve relatively few patients treated for a relatively short period of time, and therefore cannot insure the safety and effectiveness of a remedy which will be used on millions of people for many years. Often not until a remedy has been used extensively for a long period and by many physicians can its value and the possibility of adverse reactions be determined; and even then long experience is no guarantee, as the examples of bleeding and purging illustrate. With the exception of some of the errors of concept and obvious dramatic disasters, such as those occurring abruptly with BCG diethylene glycol, stalinon and hexachlorophene, it often took months or years to recognize that people were suffering, or that deaths were occurring because of ill effects of treatment. Recognition of the existence of trouble remains a major problem. Most often the first clues are reports by physicians of unusual findings — the history of x-ray exposure during infancy in children with cancer of the thyroid, sudden occurrence of unexplained or unexpected cases of poliomyelitis, jaundice, cataract, polyneuritis, phocomelia, cancer of the vagina, retrolental fibroplasia, sudden death at an early age, encephalitis. These arouse suspicion; then the tools of epidemiology are employed.

Though not related to the effects of treatment, in a simple way the epidemiological approach existed in early civilizations. Ancient Hindus noted associations between the occurrence of plague and sick and dying rats; the Athenians in classic Greece realized the immunity to recurrence of plague; the early Romans knew that cholera was spread along the trade routes.

In some instances listed here, the existence of an epidemic was obvious — the thousands of cases of hepatitis and of subacute myelo-optico-neuropathy were impossible to ignore. Large numbers of people were involved with distinctive illnesses. However, in most instances, only careful analyses and comparison revealed the presence of "a group of illnesses of similar nature, clearly in excess of normal expectation," as the American Public Health Association defines epidemic. The finding that it was beyond normal expectation to see cataract occurring in many young patients; that the rare condition of phocomelia was suddenly found in many German clinics; that there was an unexplained increase in the number of sudden deaths in children with asthma; that several cases of cancer of the vagina in adolescent girls were seen within a few years in one Boston clinic when only a few had been previously reported in the medical literature; these were the indications that "epidemics" existed. Recognition requires suspicion and knowledge of the usual frequency of the disease or condition in that population at that time, together with correlations with age, sex, timing, geography, and often other factors. The epidemic of sudden death in young asthmatics might have passed unnoticed had not an alert pediatrician, Dr. Beryl Corner, prompted by a few case reports and a rising mortality rate in young persons, carefully analyzed the mortality figures in Bristol, England, in 1966, and showed that there was an unexpectedly large number of children between the ages of ten and fourteen years of age dying from asthma. This finding was then confirmed by analyses of larger groups.

Once the existence of an epidemic is recognized, it is often difficult to detect its cause or causes. In order to avoid the many implications of the word and the extreme difficulty in proving causes, scientists use many ruses — "causal mechanisms," "factors," "relationships." The degree of frequency of association of two events — one, the disease or condition; the other, the treatment (in this context) — over and above that which might occur on a basis of chance, indicates a probability that a causal relationship may exist, but proof usually cannot be obtained by this evidence alone. Additional information, such as that derived experimentally from animals, is often useful. Even though the mechanisms of drugs in causing disease are not understood, and even without laboratory confirmation, prevention or control of the disease may be possible, as was particularly true with mercury-acrodynia and dinitrophenol-cataract; withdrawal of the drugs from the market was followed by disappearance of the epidemic.

When a condition is so rare that individual physicians may not see more than one or two cases, another method of confirming the presence of an "epidemic" is the collection of data by the establishment of registries. Winship, investigating cancer of the thyroid; Warkany, studying acrodynia; Maloney, investigating toxic cataracts; and Herbst, analyzing the problems of cancer of the vagina, wrote to many friends and colleagues for case reports and samples. More recently, this approach had been made more formal and more systematic by the formation of central registries for the accumulation of reports of drug reactions and for appropriate warning of physicians. The first such registry was established under the auspices of the American Medical Association in 1955, largely because of the efforts of Dr. Max Wintrobe in the United States. He was concerned about a serious anemia due to a failure of formation of red blood cells occurring in a few patients in 1951 who had been treated for infection with the antibiotic chloramphenicol, a widely used and effective drug. It is now estimated that only one in 60,000 to 200,000 patients receiving this drug develops severe anemia. It is a classic example of an idiosyncrasy, just as in acrodynia. In seven years, this registry received reports of 1,195 patients with blood diseases thought to be related to drug therapy. However, in only fifty-four instances were drugs thought to be possible causes. (Chloramphenicol was the most common. Its use is now advisedly restricted to the treatment of typhoid fever and certain other infections, in which it is superior to other antibiotics.) An attempt in 1961 to extend the registry to include other types of reactions to drugs failed to get backing from the American Medical Association.

The most recent specialized registry appears to be that established by Herbst and his co-workers in 1971. This is an attempt to collect as many cases as possible of cancer of the genital tract in young females. The doctor and his staff have corresponded with all obstetricians and gynecologists in the United States and three other countries. In the short span of two years they accumulated ninety-one cases, most of which confirmed their hypothesis that there is a causal relationship between stilbestrol treatment of pregnant women and the occurrence of cancer of the vagina in their offspring. This confirmation has resulted in the warning by the FDA that stilbestrol and its related forms should not be used to treat pregnant women.

After the thalidomide disaster, a registry for all suspected adverse reactions to drugs was established in the United States by the FDA. Physicians, clinical investigators, and the drug industry were required by law to report such occurrences or cases. In the United Kingdom, a limited registry for the identification of adverse drug reactions was organized in 1960 by members of the College of General Practitioners. It was a small operation, receiving only seventy-five reports during the four years of its operation. Here, as in the United States, the thalidomide catastrophe had its effect. A central registry was established, together with a Committee on Safety of Drugs, responsible to the Minister of Health. Altogether, twelve countries responded during the period from 1964 to 1967 to the public outcry resulting from the thalidomide tragedy by setting up registries for monitoring adverse reactions. The need was underlined by the lag of up to eighteen months in some countries before thalidomide was withdrawn, even after its relationship to phocomelia and polyneuritis were well established.

Co-operation on a world-wide scale began in 1958 after numerous meetings starting in 1963. A World Health Organization Drug Monitoring Centre was begun with financial help from the United States government, its membership comprising epidemiologists, statisticians, and clinical pharmacologists. Twelve nations are now collaborating, and computer programs for storage and analysis of data and special searches have been developed. Member nations not only communicate reports of suspected adverse reactions, but they also notify WHO of decisions to limit or prohibit specific drugs. An example was the notification by the Japanese government of its decision to prohibit the use of clioquinol. WHO in turn circulated the information to all member nations. Arrangements are made to signal if certain reactions or drugs are being increasingly reported. Thus, if a new and serious reaction were reported in any of the participating countries, attention would be drawn to it at an early stage, and large-scale disaster prevented.

The value of all this activity is lessened by the fact that, unfortunately, many reactions go unreported or unrecognized — particularly those occurring in hospitalized patients. This was true most recently in the sudden deaths in children with asthma (the deaths thought at first to be due to the disease, not the drug) and SMON (the disease for several years assumed to be an infectious encephalitis).

Changes in Attitude

It is evident that man's love of medicine is one of his strongest characteristics; Osler claimed it was a great feature separating man from other animals. It is also the feature responsible for the extent of harm done by many of the blunders cited here. Physicians, also, have contributed to the excessive taking of medicine by their willingness to respond and their innate need to treat. In addition, there is the enthusiasm which greets any new treatment. In the 18th century, the great clinician Heberden pointed out: "New medicines and new methods of cure always work miracles for a while." The excesses and follies resulting from the concepts of focal infection and autointoxication; the chronic use by large segments of the population, with the approval of many doctors, of mercury and silver compounds; of dinitrophenol, thalidomide, clioquinol — all for minor conditions — were responsible for most of the harm done. The dramatic nature of these tragedies has affected the attitudes of the medical profession and the public alike, for the most part in a beneficial manner. The thalidomide catastrophe was, of course, the most dramatic. (Wintrobe has spoken with bitter humour of the B.T. era — *Before Thalidomide*.) But many of the other mistakes have had their influence in producing a greater scepticism of the new and a greater respect for the hazards of all drugs. Patients as well as doctors question more often than in the past whether medicines and surgery are really necessary. Both are more cautious about the use of drugs during pregnancy and for treating trivial complaints. Additionally, physicians now more often than in the past are asking patients about drug reactions and in turn informing them about possible side-effects. Medical schools and post-graduate courses devote more time to problems and dangers of treatment. A new, highly important specialty — clinical pharmacology — has appeared partly as a result. The pharmaceutical industry itself has become more cautious, less flamboyant. The change in attitude has been a limited but healthy antidote to our over-selling of therapeutic "miracles." Excesses are still with us on the part of the profession as well as the public. In 1970 Wade wrote, "The dawn of concern about adverse reactions to drugs has broken; its light has yet to shine in every corner."

Finally — although it is often overlooked — there has developed a healthy humility. The doctrine of professorial infallibility, the arrogant, authoritarian, autocratic attitude so common among successful academic physicians and surgeons, is disappearing in the western world and is being replaced by a willingness to submit all treatments to critical tests. Errors of concept vigorously promulgated by zealous, influential enthusiasts should also have less chance in the future.

One of the major problems and hazards resulting from the pharmacological revolution in the past three decades is the confusion caused by the sheer number of available drugs, many of which are closely related in their action. There are now more than 22,000 prescription preparations, the so-called ethical pharmaceuticals, on the market in the United States, many of them worthless. In addition, there are thousands of proprietary drugs, mostly combinations, which are sold without prescriptions. These, of course, include sedatives, headache remedies, cold remedies, laxatives, cough medicines and pain relievers. All too many of these are ineffective. Many are effective but have adverse side effects, and do not cure the basic disease; the inclusion of antibiotics in proprietary cold remedies is an example of this.

Several hundred new drugs come onto the market each year, but only a few are really important and represent true advances in treatment. (Miracles do not occur even once a year!) Most of the preparations represent no improvement over the old remedies, yet such is the eagerness of the public to receive, and of the physician to prescribe, what is new because it is new, that they are readily sold. Clearly, it is impossible for any physician to become familiar and at ease with the use of more than a limited number of remedies. Fortunately doctors can give their patients excellent care employing only a few dozen drugs. With few exceptions, it is not advisable or necessary to give more than one drug in any preparation. Yet a large majority of the new products on the market each year are new mixtures of old drugs packaged more attractively and given new names. Several of the examples cited in this group of errors illustrate this point well: thalidomide was incorporated in over 100 mixtures; phenacetin is rarely sold alone and is found in dozens of combinations sold in most countries; aminopyrine is still to be found in many headache remedies and is often prescribed and used unsuspectingly by physicians and public alike; clioquinol, according to the Japanese physicians, was found in 184 different remedies. Not only does this use of many combinations cause confusion, but it also prevents or delays productive action when adverse effects occur, because physicians are frequently unaware of the contents of these mixtures.

Confusion is also increased, because most drugs are given proprietary names by their manufacturers, who make every effort to promote their products under their own names. Thus a single chemical substance will often be marketed under half a dozen names. Teachers and textbooks alike urge the profession to use the official non-proprietary generic names, and the FDA now requires the official name to be included on the label. But the problem remains largely unsolved.

In England and the United States, the requirements regarding the issuance of an entirely new drug demand many safeguards. However, as yet no satisfactory way has been evolved to get rid of old drugs which are without value and are sometimes hazardous. The FDA is making strong efforts in this direction, but there is much opposition on the part of the public and many doctors, as well as the pharmaceutical houses.

Changes in Legislation

During the present century, most industrialized countries have come to recognize the need to regulate the manufacture, sale, and use of drugs, and have passed legislation for this purpose, most of it in the past decade. This necessity has been largely due to sheer numbers of effective and potentially toxic drugs which have become available during this period; it is estimated that nine-tenths of the thousands of presently used drugs have arrived on the market since 1930.

The mistakes and accidents described here were responsible for the passage of much of this legislation. The early problems with the manufacture, sterilization, and purity of vaccines and biological products resulting in the Lübeck disaster, and the recurrent epidemics of hepatitis following the use of other vaccines stimulated laws and regulations for the standardization and inspection of these complex agents. The diethylene glycol (Elixir of Sulfanilamide) and the Stalinon poisonings aroused the profession and the public to the realization that products need to be tested for toxicity before they are released for human use. Most recently there has been a tendency, brought on in part by the problems with phenacetin, in the United States, England, and Sweden, to limit the excessive use and misuse of sedatives, sleeping pills, tranquilizers, and analgesics, by restricting their sale to pharmacies, or by requiring that they be sold by prescription only.

But it was the shock of the thalidomide catastrophe more than any other single event which made the profession and public alike aware that all effective drugs are potentially toxic and that controls are required. The resulting restrictive legislation, which varies widely from country to country, has done much to reduce the risk of widespread disasters and to improve both animal and clinical testing. Most industrial countries now require quality control in the manufacture, packaging, and storage of all forms of medicines, and insist on both animal and clinical trials. In the toxicity tests on animals, experiments for possible carcinogenic and teratogenic effects are usually mandatory. In many countries, some proof is required that a new drug be shown to be effective for indications recommended. In the capitalist countries, the burden of proof of quality, safety, and efficacy rests with the manufacturer.

The most restrictive legislation is found in the United States, the largest producer of all types of drugs. James Young, an American historian, has termed the important restrictive federal legislation governing food, drugs, and cosmetics in the United States the result of "compromise, crusading, and catastrophe." The first important omnibus bill passed in 1906 was the result of sixteen years of negotiations. The catastrophe leading to its passage was the precipitous fall in the sale of meat, resulting from the exposures of the grim practices of meat packers in Upton Sinclair's muckraking novel, *The Jungle*. This bill forbade mislabelling and adulteration.

The second omnibus bill was passed in 1938, largely as a result of the diethylene glycol, "Elixir of Sulfanilamide", tragedy, in which there occurred seventy-three deaths, mostly of children. This calamity produced an unusually strong public reaction. Among other things, this bill established testing for toxicity, and it also provided effective control over false advertising. Both of these provisions later supported Dr. Frances Kelsey, acting on behalf of the FDA, in her successful efforts to withhold thalidomide from the market. In the spring of 1961, she wrote, "It is the responsibility of this Administration to be satisfied that a new drug has been demonstrated to be safe before it may be released for general marketing in the U.S." She states further, "In the consideration of an application for a new drug, the burden of proof that the drug causes side-effects does not lie with this Administration. The burden of proof that the drug is safe, which must include adequate studies of all the manifestations of toxicity which medical or clinical experience suggests, lies with the applicant." This law and the alertness of Dr. Kelsey saved the United States from the catastrophe suffered by many other countries, none of which had such restrictive legislation. It has been argued that it was only a matter of luck and bureaucratic procrastination. Undoubtedly, luck played a part. But two factors unrelated to bureaucratic procrastination delayed the acceptance of thalidomide for general use: the lack of adequate planned controlled clinical trials performed by qualified investigators — most reports were hardly better than testimonials — and the early reports of polyneuritis in patients using the drug for prolonged periods.

The third major law, the Drug Amendment for 1962, was vigorously contested but passed as a result of the reaction by the public and the U.S. Senate to the thalidomide catastrophe. This legislation, which appears to be more restrictive than that of any other country, was fought by the drug industry, the American Medical Association, and the press. The fascinating story of the political manoeuvring has been told in detail by Harris, in the *Real Voice*. The main provisions of the bill related to the requirement that manufacturers demonstrate that a drug is effective as well as safe. In addition, much more rigid safety controls were instituted, demanding extensive animal experimentation before a drug could be released for clinical trials on human beings. (Testing of chronic toxicity in animals had not been done with thalidomide.) Also, manufacturers were required to provide generic names on all labels and to include information on side effects, contra-indications, and effectiveness. (Chemie Grunenthal claimed that thalidomide was

160

"completely innocuous," "completely atoxic," and the best drug to be administered to pregnant and nursing mothers.)

Many other western countries, reacting in similar fashion, have passed legislation since 1962 controlling the release of new drugs, but none have reacted as strongly as has the United States. Surprisingly enough, the two countries who suffered the most, West Germany and Japan, have passed the least restrictive laws.

Many scientists and physicians have felt that there is overreaction and that the present laws in the United States are much too restrictive, delaying or even preventing valuable drugs from reaching the market. The editor of the American *Yearbook of Drug Therapy* in 1973 stated, "The point may be approaching where we are doing more harm than good by our restrictive policies." Visscher, the American physiologist, in a letter to *Science,* in 1967, expressed concern about "harm to the public welfare" due to the regulations. He admits that "great caution and exhaustive study of all possible ill effects" of a new drug should be made before releasing it for general sale. He objects to the "excessively elaborate" toxicity studies in animals required prior to approval of limited clinical studies, and suggests that lives are being lost by the delay in making valuable drugs available, and by the inhibition of research. It is true that the present formal requirements for approval for general use of a single new drug are formidable. They are complex and require the investment of hundreds of thousands of dollars, large technical staffs, and the availability in sufficient numbers of both healthy volunteers and patients with certain diseases. A delay of several years before a drug is put on the market is the inevitable consequence. A useful, effective but non-essential cardiovascular drug — propanolol — was in general use in England for five years before it was released in the United States. The legislation appears to have resulted in a smaller number of new drugs being marketed each year in the United States. There is general agreement that the purposes of the FDA are good, but that its function and flexibility need to be improved so that there will be fewer delays and the rules can be revised in response to new scientific ideas and technical findings.

Max Tishler, former President for Research at Merck, Sharp and Dohme, in 1973 listed some of the effective drugs available for several years in other countries before the FDA permitted their sale in the United States. In addition to propanolol, the list included furosemide, a highly effective and widely used diuretic; and ampicillin, one of the broad-spectrum antibiotics. In England, furosemide was available for five years and ampicillin for two years before either could be purchased in the United States. Tishler makes the useful suggestion that a running account be kept of specific drugs available in other countries which cannot be obtained in the United States. He argues that the major emphasis of the FDA is to protect the public from potential harm rather than to accelerate the availability of helpful drugs for the sick.

The important question is whether in our efforts to insure safety we are losing more than we are gaining. Absolute safety is unattainable; there is a price for progress.

Nevertheless, the drug industry in the United States continues to flourish. The critics do not cite any examples of life-saving, essential drugs (for which there are no substitutes) available in other countries with less stringent laws but which are not yet allowed in the United States. Finally, the fact that the three great drug-induced epidemics of the last decade — phocomelia and polyneuritis, sudden death in young asthmatics, and subacute myelo-opticoneuropathy, which involved more than 30,000 people, all occurred in countries with laws much more lax, cannot be overlooked.

In the United Kingdom before the thalidomide disaster, any company could produce and market a new medicine, no matter how inadequately tested; but in the wake of the tragedy, action was rapidly taken. In December 1963 the Ministry of Health established the Safety of Drugs Committee. This was a small, distinguished, able, professional group, with no legal power but with great moral persuasion, serving voluntarily. They screened the evidence of toxicity tests and clinical trials submitted by the manufacturers of all new drugs, laying down standards and making recommendations. This simple arrangement functioned remarkably well, and the sixty-odd new drugs each year were cleared for release in about three months after receipt of the application. (Most, of course, required one or more years to be tested.) Little or no restriction was placed on proprietary drugs such as cold remedies and laxatives, thought to be harmless. In 1969 new legislation, the

Medical Act, was passed. This extended the functions of the Committee and gave it legal power. Controls were placed over advertising and promotional material. These powers enabled the Committee to issue warnings and force changes in advertising claims in connection with the pressurized aerosol bronchodilators, clioquinol, and phenacetin, when disasters resulted from their misuse.

Gain in Scientific Knowledge

Not the least of the effects of the mistakes discussed in this book has been the positive increase of scientific knowledge. The results of irradiation of the thymus demonstrated that, in man, the cancer-producing effects of x-ray could be delayed for eight to ten years. The experience with contaminated yellow fever vaccine showed that viral hepatitis (previously called catarrhal jaundice) could be transmitted by any material contaminated with human serum from a donor who had had the disease recently, and the virus was remarkably resistant and a serious hazard whenevr injected alive into the human body. Thalidomide proved to be the most potent teratogenic agent for man and monkey yet known, thereby expanding concepts of embryology and facilitating the study of the mechanisms by which congenital malformations are produced.

The recent proven association between the administration of stilbestrol to pregnant mothers and the development of vaginal cancer in their daughters ten to twenty years later disclosed two important possibilities. The first was that this drug therapy could be carcinogenic. Previously, with the exception of radioactive material, only arsenical salts, coal tars, and smoking were known to cause cancer in man. (They produced a dermatitis which was sometimes followed by the development of low-grade skin cancers.) The second was the possibility that cells potentially capable of becoming cancerous may lie dormant for many years until stimulated by the hormonal influences producing the many changes of sexual maturation during adolescence.

The damage to the eyes of premature babies produced by oxygen administration during the first weeks of life taught that high concentrations of oxygen in the blood have a specific destructive

163

effect on growing blood vessels in the retina, and led in turn to careful monitoring of oxygen tensions in the blood of premature babies and generally better management in premature nurseries.

The sudden deaths in young asthmatics associated with the use of isoproterenol inhalants led to the experiments in dogs which indicated that under conditions of lowered blood oxygen concentrations, the circulatory system is particularly vulnerable to this and to similar drugs.

Value of Previous Experience

> Those who have no knowledge of the past are doomed to repeat its mistakes.
>
> Santayana

Another of the lessons taught is that we need to know of the previous experience of others. Work in the library should precede experiment. Warkany has convincingly told how the astute clinician of a hundred years ago would have recognized the signs and symptoms of acrodynia as mercury poisoning due to chronic use of calomel. Classic descriptions of argyria resulting from prolonged use of silver preparations were written two centuries ago, yet many physicians ignored the hazard.

The outbreak of 28,000 cases of hepatitis among U.S. soldiers in 1942 was a strong reminder of the need for a knowledge of medical literature. Three million men were immunized in a period of fifteen months. At first an association between the vaccination for yellow fever and hepatitis was not suspected, though it was recognized that this was one possibility among many. Yet knowledge of past experience would have made it clear that an association was probable. In 1883, one of the first large-scale drug catastrophes occurred at a shipyard in Bremen. From one lot of vaccine, 1,281 men were vaccinated against smallpox, with glycerinated human serum; 191 subsequently developed jaundice. Detailed reports of hepatitis and jaundice among persons vaccinated for yellow fever in England in 1937 and in Brazil in 1936, 1937, 1939, 1940, and 1941 had appeared in readily available medical journals. A total of 1,072 cases had occurred during 1940 and 1941. Further, it was clearly recognized that the use of human serum was a likely causal factor and that the disease was of an infectious nature. (At that time, the nature of viral hepatitis was not known.) In retrospect, the lesson did not seem to have been learned from these previous epidemics.

Over a sixteen-month period, four and a half million American soldiers and sailors were immunized. Only a fraction of these men were sent to areas of the world where yellow fever was a threat. In the light of the knowledge available to the armed forces medical corps, it seems that a smaller trial could have been made, and that the risks had not been appreciated.

The two large mass poisonings of the century — those caused by stalinon and by diethylene glycol (the solvent in Elixir of Sulfanilamide) — could easily have been avoided had the pharmacists who formulated and marketed these products read the easily available recent accounts of their toxicity in animals.

Again, in retrospect, it became obvious that the masculinizing effects on the female fetus produced by the synthetic progestins should have been anticipated by the obstetricians prescribing the drugs for pregnant women. Several years before the drugs were first used on patients, two well-known French endocrinologists had demonstrated similar adverse effects in rabbits and had warned specifically about these hazards if the drugs were used to prevent spontaneous abortion in human beings. Yet there is no evidence that either the pharmaceutical firms advertising the drugs or the physicians prescribing them were aware of these warnings.

In the future, the ease of retrieval of such information when stored appropriately in the memory banks of a computer system may prevent similar mistakes.

Conclusion

Considering the multitude of effective treatments made available in the present century, it is not surprising that some major errors have been committed; in many ways it is surprising that there have not been more. However, it is often assumed that they were for the most part inevitable or unavoidable. Clearly, this was not the case. Most of the suffering and deaths were avoidable and were due to two basic causes: premature release for general use of various forms of treatment before they had been adequately tested on both animals and human beings; and excessive use of remedies often non-essential or ineffective. The extent of the harm could often have been much reduced by earlier recognition brought about by monitoring.

With respect to the first of these causes, it is clear that scientific testing of all forms of therapy is the best protection against disaster, and the best way to determine efficacy. But most forms of treatment were discarded because of reasons other than evidence furnished by empiric animal or clinical trials. Bleeding by venesection, arterial puncture, or the use of leeches became less popular and less frequently used because of the comparisons made by P.C.A. Louis in the 1830s, but they were not given up until the present century. As late as 1912, in the eighth edition of his textbook of medicine, Osler, the most influential teacher of his time and an admirer of Louis, still advised venesection for the early treatment of pneumonia, if the patients were "young and robust." The use of purgatives and enemas for constipation, and to rid the body of intestinal poisons, as we have seen, extended into the middle of the present century. Both of these treatments, which now appear to have done little good and much harm to many hundreds of thousands, were widely used for many diseases for more than two thousand years. The test of time failed miserably to eliminate them. They were finally abandoned because of better understanding of the physiology and the wisdom of the human body.

Similarly, new knowledge and improved techniques in bacteriology and immunology were more responsible for discarding the concepts of focal infection and vaccine therapy than were the few clinical trials made. More careful anatomical and pathological observations and measurements provided the evidence leading to exposure of the concept of status thymicolymphaticus. Finally, bitter experience alone was often sufficient, as in the attempts to revascularize the brain and to glue fractures, and in the many iatrogenic diseases produced by drugs. The tragedy was that in most cases many years elapsed before the errors were recognizd; appropriate trials performed early could have prevented untold suffering caused by the treatments. As Hill points out: "The history of medicine abounds with remedies that were long and widely used before falling into disrepute and vanishing. A designed test might have greatly hastened their fall from favour and have thereby encouraged the search for something better."

In this century, two-thirds of the major errors presented here could have been avoided if the treatments had not been prematurely released and advised for general use before they had been adequately tested and tried on animals and Man; either lack of efficacy or important harmful effects would have been demonstrated. Most, if not all, of the treatments resulting from the errors of concept could have been so exposed by appropriate trials.

The uselessness or the harmful side effects of more than half the drugs (such as thallium, dinitrophenol, stalinon, triparanol, the progestins, gold, and probably aminorex and thalidomide) would have been made apparent. Two of the laboratory mistakes — the use of the solvent diethylene glycol, and of the enteric-coated potassium chloride tablets — would have been avoided had suitable animal trials been made before the general release of the medications. Generalizations are more difficult with respect to the overdoses, though it is obvious in retrospect that, had appropriate animal tests been performed, the damage done by giving too much oxygen to premature infants and by advising the prolonged use of clioquinol need not have resulted. Controlled clinical trials of high doses of vitamin D would have almost surely demonstrated its inefficaciousness in the treatment of tuberculosis, psoriasis, and arthritis, even if they had not exposed its toxiciy.

Wih regard to the second major basic cause of these errors, the excessive use of forms of treatment often non-essential or ineffective in the maintenance of health or their misuse for trivial complaints, appear to account for a third of the thirty-two major errors analyzed here. These include: laxatives (cathartics, including calomel and colonic irrigations for "regularity" and to avoid auto-intoxication); phenacetin pain and headache relievers (consumed not only to relieve pain and discomfort, but also to permit the patient "to feel better"); clioquinol (used by millions of Japanese for months and years to "regulate" their intestinal functions); silver compounds such as argyrol employed as antiseptics by painting the throat, irrigating the sinuses, or given as enemas or douches; mercury-containing teething powders for infants; reducing drugs (dinitrophenal and aminorex); the sedative and hypnotic, thalidomide; aerosol bronchodilators for relief of asthma; high-potency vitamin D compounds; and extraction of tonsils as a general health measure and cold preventive. Most of the drugs were used daily for the flimsiest of reasons for periods of months or years. Almost all were freely available to the general public for purchase over the counter in a variety of stores as well as in pharmacies. The remedies were used in the vain search for health and well-being, in the foolish but persistent belief that health and well-being can be purchased and maintained by medication or surgery. With the important excepions of preventive inoculations for specific infectious diseases, and judicious use of vitamins at certain periods of life, this is seldom true.

Benjamin Franklin's observation — "Nothing is more fatal to health than an overcare of it" — remains valid. The truth is that the rules of health are simple and are related to diet, exercise, the avoidance of smoking and excessive use of alcohol. These rules improve our chances, but do not allow us to avoid most of the catastrophic diseases which threaten us all — cancer, stroke, heart attack, mental disorders. One shrewd observer has noted that in the United States, by and large, those who have the best medical care and advice readily available to them at the least expense are the families of the specialists in internal medicine. These families use less medicine and undergo less surgery on the whole than any other group, rich or poor. Yet, when they are truly ill, they readily receive effective, often hazardous drugs, and are operated on quickly if they require surgery. The lesson is that stated by Osler over a half-century ago: "One of the first duties of the physician is to educate the masses not to take medicine." One must also, in fairness, add that many physicians need to be educated not to prescribe unnecessarily.

What of the present and the future? This review does not help to indicate specifically the errors we are committing now, nor what treatment disasters will occur in the future, but it strongly suggests that they have not ended. The three major epidemics resulting from the use of thalidomide, aerosol bronchodilators, and clioquinol, as well as the minor ones involving the use of coated potassium chloride, triparanol, aminorex, the progestins, and phenacetin, are all too recent. But past experience does offer clues as to the type of errors to anticipate. These will probably result from: 1) inadequately planned and executed animal tests, or the lack of controlled clinical trials of new methods, new drugs, new operations (it is obvious that there are insufficient facilities and trained personnel to carry out the ones needed now), before release for general use; or 2) excessive and foolish use of unnecessary remedies. There remains far too much demand for these on the part of the public, and too much willingness on the part of the doctors to prescribe. The imaginary invalid is still with us.

In addition, it is apparent that we can anticipate the occurrence of late adverse side effects of drugs — even ones which have been in use for years. Unless the present lack of adequate records of the use of drugs for individual patients is corrected, the recognition of these late effects will continue to be delayed.

The "doctor's dilemma" is not the choice of whom to save, as in Shaw's play. Rather it is the dilemma that every doctor faces daily, with varying success, of how to treat and help without harming. The Hippocratic admonition, "first do no harm," cannot strictly apply. Risks must be taken if benefits are to be maximal. Harm will often occur, and constant vigilance is required to keep it minimal. Few risks are justified when the illness is minor and self-limited.

Major risks may be justified when the illness is major, death likely, and no simple effective treatment is available.

The Greek word *pharmakon* is translated "drug," or "medicine." But Henry Sigerist, the medical historian, points out that in Homeric times the word referred to a talisman which could be used for good or evil — to turn men into swine, to poison them, or to effect a cure. All effective drugs and surgical procedures have the potential for harm as well as benefit. Technically, we now possess a capacity for good and evil on a world-wide scale — a scale never attained before. It will take all our efforts to keep the *pharmakon* a talisman preponderantly good.

References

Chapter Two   Laboratory Mistakes and Accidents

Lübeck Disaster — BCG

Foster, W. D. 1970, *A history of medical bacteriology and immunology*. London: Wm. Heinemann Medical Books Ltd., p. 158.

Henderson, D. A.; Witte, J. J.; Morris, L.; and Langmuir, A. D. 1964. Paralytic disease associated with oral polio vaccines. *JAMA* 190:41.

Wilson, G. S. 1967. *Hazards of Immunization*. London: Athlone Press, p. 66.

Diethylene Glycol — Elixir of Sulfanilamide

Journal of the American Medical Association. 1937*a*. Deaths following elixir of sulfanilamide — Massengill. Editorial 109:1367.

———. 1937*b*. Report on federal legislation relating to foods, drugs, diagnostic and theraputic devices and cosmetics. Editorial 109:738. tic and therapeutic devices and cosmetics. Editorial 109:738.

Geiling, E. M. K.; and Cannon, P. R. 1938. Pathologic effects of elixir of sulfanilamide (diethylene glycol) poisoning: clinical and experimental correlation: final report. *JAMA* 111:919.

Lynch, K. M. 1938. Diethylene glycol poisoning in the human. *South. Med. J.* 31:134.

Von Oettingen, W. F.; and Jirouch, E. A. 1931. Acute toxicity of diethylene glycol. *J. of Pharm. and Exp. Med.* 42:355.

Contaminated Yellow Fever Vaccine

Journal of the American Medical Association. 1942. Outbreak of jaundice in the army (circular letter no. 95, Office of Surgeon General). Editorial 120:51-2.

Fox, J. P.; Manso, C.; Penna, H. A., and Madureira, P. 1942. Observations on occurrence of icterus in Brazil following vaccination against yellow fever. *Am. J. Hyg.* 36:68.

Rhodes, A. J.; and Van Rooyen, C. E. 1958. *Textbook of Virology.* 3rd ed. Baltimore: Williams and Wilkins Co. p. 313.

Sawyer, W. A.; Meyer, K. F.; Eaton, M. D.; Bauer, J. H.; Putnam, P.; and Schwentker, F. F. 1944. Jaundice in army personnel in the western region of the United States and its relation to vaccination against yellow fever. *Am. J. Hyg.* 39:337.

Strode, G. K., ed. 1951. *Yellow Fever.* New York: McGraw-Hill. pp. 36-7.

Turner, R. H. *et al.* 1944. Some clinical studies of acute hepatitis occurring in soldiers after inoculation with yellow fever vaccine with especial consideration of severe attacks. *Ann. Int. Med.* 20:193.

Cutter Incident — Polio Vaccine

Boyd, T. E. 1957. *A biography of poliomyelities.* N.Y. Acad. of Sci. special publication. 5:39.

World Health Organization. 1958. *The First Ten Years of the World Health Organization.* Geneva.

Nathanson, N.; and Langmuir, A. D. 1963. Poliomyelitis following formaldehyde-inactivated poliovirus vaccination in the United States during the spring of 1955. *Am. J. Hyg.* 78:16.

Scheele, L. A.; and Shannon, J. A. 1955. Public health implications in a program against poliomyelities. *JAMA* 158:1249.

New York Academy of Science. 1960. Symposium: inactivation of viruses. *Ann. N.Y. Acad. of Sci.* 83:513.

Coated Potassium Chloride Tablets

Baker, D. R.; Schrader, W. H.; and Hitchcock, C. R. 1964. Small-bowel ulceration apparently associated with thiazide and potassium therapy. *JAMA* 190:586.

Binns, T. B. 1965. Stockholm: Proceedings of European Society for Study of Drug Toxicity.

Boley, S. J.; Schultz, L.; Kruger, H.; Schwartz, S.; Elguezbal, A.; and Allen, A. C. 1965. Experimental evaluation of thiazides and potassium as a cause of small bowel ulcer. *JAMA* 192:763.

Doll, R. 1971. Unwanted effects of drugs. *Br. Med. Bull.* 27:25

Journal of the American Medical Association. 1965. Small bowel ulceration: in pursuit of an etiology. Editorial 191:668.

Lawrason, F. D.; Alpert, F.; Mohr, F. L.; and McMahon, F. G. 1965. Ulcerative-obstructive lesions of the small intestine. *JAMA* 191:641.

Morgenstern, L.; Freilich, M.; and Panish, J. F. 1965. The circumferential small-bowel ulcer. *JAMA* 191:637.

Raff, L. E. 1967. Enteric coated potassium chloride tablets and ulcer of the small intestine. *Acta. Chir. Scand. Suppl.* 374:197.

Hexachlorophene

American Academy of Pediatrics Committee on Fetus and Newborn 1972. Hexachlorophene and skin care of newborn infants. *Ped.* 49:625.

Plueckhahn, V. D. 1973. Hexachlorophene and skin care of newborn infants. *Drugs* 5:97.

Chapter Three   Side Effects of Drugs

Teething Powders and Laxatives — Pink Disease

Warkany, J.; and Hubbard, D. M. 1948. Mercury in the urine of children with acrodynia. *Lancet* 1:829.

―――. 1951. Adverse mercurial reactions in the form of acrodynia and other related conditions. *Am. J. Dis. Child.* 81:335.

Warkany, J. 1966. Acrodynia — postmortem of a disease. *Am. J. Dis.*

Silver Antiseptics — Blue-Grey Skin

DiPalma, J. R., ed. 1965. *Drill's Pharmacology in Medicine.* New York: McGraw-Hill, pp. 1648-9.

Engley, F. B., Jr. 1950. Evaluation of mercurial compounds as antiseptics. *Ann. N.Y. Acad. Sci.* 53:197.

Gaul, L. E.; and Staud, A. H. 1935. Clinical spectroscopy: 70 cases of argyria. *JAMA* 104:1387.

Levine, S. A.; and Smith, J. A. 1942. Argyria confused with heart disease. *Am. Heart J.* 23:739.

Stillians, A. W. 1937. Argyria. *Arch. Dermat and Syph.* 35:67.

A Depilatory — Poisoning and Death

Bedford, G. V. 1928. Depilation with thallium acetate in treatment of ringworm of scalp in children. *Canad. M.A.J.* 19:660.

DiPalma, J. R., ed. 1965. *Drill's Pharmacology in Medicine.* New York: McGraw-Hill. pp. 1133, 1272.

Journal of the American Medical Association. 1929. Thallium poisoning. Editorial 92:1865.

Gleich, M. 1931. Thallium acetate poisoning in the treatment of ringworm of the scalp. *JAMA* 97:851.

Grulee, C. G. Jr.; and Clark, E. H. 1951. Thallotoxicosis (from eating rodenticide) in preschool nursery; 4 cases. *Am. J. Dis. Child.* 81:47.

Grunfeld, O.; Aldana, L.; and Hinostroza, G. 1963. Radiological aspects of thallium poisoning. *Radiol.* 80:847.

Heyroth, F. F. 1947. Thallium: a review and summary of the medical literature. *Pub. Health Rep.,* Suppl. 197.

Ingram, J. T. 1932. Thallium acetate in treatment of ringworm of scalp. *Brit. Med. J.* 1:8.

Munch, J. C. 1934. Human thallotoxicosis. *JAMA* 102:1929.

A Headache Powder and Pain Reliever —
Disease of the White Blood Cells

Dameshek, W.; and Ingall, M. 1931. Agranulocytosis (malignant neutropenia), *Amer. J. Med. Sci.* 181:502.

Discombe, G. 1952. Agranulocytosis caused by amidopyrine. *Brit. Med. J.* 1:1270.

Hart, P. W. 1973. Drug induced agranulocytosis. In *Blood disorders due to drugs,* Girdwood, R. H., ed. Amsterdam: Exerpta Medica. p. 147.

Huguley, C. M., Jr. 1966. Hematalogical reactions. *JAMA* 196:408.

Huguley, C. M.; Erslev, A. J.; and Begsagel, D. E. 1961. Drug-related blood discrasias. *JAMA* 177:23.

Kracke, R. R.; and Parker, F. P. 1934. The etiology of granulopenia (agranulocytosis) with particular reference to drugs containing the benezene ring. *Am. J. Clin. Path.* 4:453.

Mosbech, J.; and Riis, P. 1960. Mortality from agranulocytosis in Denmark. *Acta. Med. Scand.* 166:343.

Sturgis, C. C. 1955. *Hematology,* 2nd ed. Springfield, Ill.: C. C. Thomas. p. 982.

Wade, O. L. 1970. *Adverse Reactions to Drugs.* London: Wm. Heinemann Medical Books. Ltd. p. 6.

Gold in Tuberculosis — Disease of the White Blood Cells

Foster, W. D. 1970. *A History of Medical Bacteriology and Immunology.* London: Wm. Heinemann Medical Books Ltd. p. 204.

Hart, P. D. 1946. Chemotherapy of tuberculosis: research in the past 100 years. *Brit. Med. J.* 2:805.

Hartfall, S. J.; Garland, H. G.; and Goldie, W. 1937. Gold treatment of arthritis; review of 900 cases. *Lancet* 2:838.

Mollgaard, H. 1925. The sanocrysin treatment of tuberculosis. *Brit. Med. J.* 1:643.

Peters, B. A.; and Short, C. 1935. Gold treatment of tuberculosis: a statistical study. *Lancet* 2:11.

Rest, A. 1943. Gold therapy in tuberculosis. *Am. Rev. of Tuberc.* 47:406

Medical Research Council. 1926. Second report by the Medical Research Council. Gold treatment of tuberculosis. *Brit. Med. J.* 2:158.

Scadding, J. G. 1960. Clinical aspects of controlled trials. In *Controlled Clinical Trials,* Hill, A. B., ed. Oxford: Blackwell Scientific Publications, p. 52.

Sutherland, I. 1960. Pulmonary tuberculosis. In *Controlled Clinical Trials,* Hill, A. B., ed. Oxford: Blackwell Scientific Publications. p. 47.

Wells, H. G. 1932. The chemotherapy of tuberculosis. *Yale J. Biol. and Med.* 4:611.

A Reducing Pill — Cataract

Journal of the American Medical Association. 1936. Dilex Redusols. Article 106:1587.

―――. 1935. German Federal Bureau of Health. Article 104:1260.

―――. 1935. Council on Pharmacy and Chemistry. Article 104:1998.

Cutting, W. C.; Mehrtens, H. G., and Tainter, M. L. 1933. Action and uses of dinitrophenol. *JAMA* 101:193.

Journal of the American Medical Asociation. 1933. The toxicity of dinitrophenol. Editorial 101:1080.

Heitch, J. M.; and Schwartz, W. F. 1936. Late toxic results, including dermatitis exfoliativa, from "slim" (dinitrophenol). *JAMA* 106:2130.

Horner, W. D. 1942. Dinitrophenol and its relation to formation of cataract. *Arch. Ophth.* 27:1097.

Journal of the American Medical Association. 1934. Sales barred DNT. Medical News 103:1243.

―――. 1936. Treatment of obesity. Queries 107:1490.

Silver, S. 1934. A new danger in dinitrophenol therapy — agranulocytosis with fatal outcome. *JAMA* 103:1059.

Tainter, M. L.; Stockton, A. B.; and Cutting, W. C. 1933. Use of dinitrophenol in obesity and related conditions. *JAMA* 101:1474.

Synthetic Hormones — Masculinization of Daughters

Briebart, S.; Bongiovanni, A. M.; Eberlein, W. R. 1963. Progestins and skeletal maturation. *New Eng. J. Med.* 268:255.

Cohen, R. L. 1966. Experimental and clinical chemoteratogenesis. *Adv. Pharmacol.* 4:263.

Courrier, R.; and Jost, A. 1942. *Intersexualité foetale provoquée par la pregneninolone au cours de la grossesse. Compt. rend. Soc. de Biol.* 136:395.

Goldzieher, J. W. 1964. Double-blind trial of a progestin in habitual abortion. *JAMA* 188:651.

Grumbach, M. M.; Ducharme, J. R.; and Moloshok, R. E. 1959. On the fetal masculinizing action of certain oral progestins. *J. of Clin. Endocrin.* 19:1369.

Hellman, L. M.; and Pritchard, J. A. 1971. In *William's Obstetrics,* 14th ed. London: Butterworths. pp. 507-11.

Jones, H. W., Jr. 1957. Female hermaphroditism without virilization. *Obst. and Gynec. Surv.* 12:433.

Jones, H. W., Jr.; and Wilkins, L. 1960. The genital anomaly associated with prenatal exposure to progestogens. *Fertil. and Steril.* 11:148.

Shearman, R. P.; and Garrett, W. J. 1963. Double-blind study of the effect of 17—hydroxyprogesterone caproate on abortion rate. *Brit. Med. J.* 5326:292.

Voorhess, M. J. 1967. Masculinization of the female fetus associated with norethindrone — mestranol therapy during pregnancy. *J. Pediat.* 171:128.

Wilkins, L. 1950. *Diagnosis and Treatment of Endocrine Disorders in Childhood and Adolescence.* Springfield, Ill.: C. C. Thomas.

———. 1960. Masculinization of female fetus due to use of orally given progestins. *JAMA* 172:1028.

Wilkins, L.; Jones, H. W., Jr.; Holman, G. H.; and Stempfel, R. S., Jr. 1958. Masculinization of the female fetus associated with administration of oral and intra-muscular progestins during gestation: nonadrenal female pseudohermaphrodism. *J. Clin. Endocrin. and Metab.* 18:559.

Wilson, J. G. 1973. Present status of drugs as teratogen in man. *Teratology* 7:1.

A Treatment for Boils — Encephalitis

Fontan, A.; Pesme, P.; and Verger, P. 1955. Ocular complications of stalinon intoxication. *Bull. Soc. Ophth. Fr.* 1-2:123.

Stoner, H. B.; Barnes, J. M.; and Duff, J. I. 1955. Toxicity, alkyl tin compounds. *Br. J. Pharmacol.* 10:16.

Wade, O. L. 1970. *Adverse Reactions to Drugs.* London: Wm. Heinemann Medical Books Ltd. p. 10.

Bergen, S. B.; and Van Itallie, T. E. 1963. Approaches to the treatment of hypercholesteremia. *Ann. Intern. Med.* 58:355.

Chiu, G. C. 1961. Mode of action of cholesterol-lowering agents — a critique of facts and theories. *Archiv. Int. Med.* 108:717.

Goodman, D. S.; Avigan, J. *International Pharmocological Meeting,* vol. 2, eds. E. C. Herning, P. Lindgren. Oxford: Pergamon Press.

Kirby, T. J. 1967. Cataracts produced by triparanol (MER-29). *Trans. Amer. Optical Soc.* 65:494.

Medical Letter. Jan. 1962. MER-29 and warnings on new drugs. *Med. Letter* No. 2:5 4:5.

Laughlin, R. C.; and Carey, T. F. 1962. Cataracts in patients treated with triparanol. *JAMA* 181:339.

Minton, L. R.; and Bounds, G. W. 1963. Ophthalmologic findings in patients with ectodermal side-effects while on MER-29. *Am. J. Ophth.* 55:787.

Mintz, M. 1967. *By Prescription Only.* Boston: Houghton Mifflin Co.

Modell, W. 1967. In *Drug Responses in Man.* Wolstenholme, G.; and Porter, R. J. and A., eds. London: Churchill Ltd. pp. 2, 13.

Perry, H. O.; Winkelmann, R. K.; Achor, R. W.; and Kirby, T. J., Jr. 1962. Side effects of triparanol therapy. *Amer. J. Med. Sci.* 244:556.

Stamler, J. 1967. *Lectures on preventive cardiology.* London: Grune & Stratton Inc. N.Y. pp. 210, 220.

Wright, I. S. 1960. In *Progress in Cardiovascular Disease 2 (No. 6)* Princeton, N.J.: Proc. Conference on MER-29 (Triparanol).

Thalidomide — Deformed Children, Polyneuritis

Cohen, S. 1962. Thalidomide polyneuropathy. *N. Eng. J. Med.* 266:1268.

Delahunt, C. S.; and Lassen, L. J. 1964. Thalidomide syndrome in monkeys. *Science* 146:1300.

Hafstrom, T. 1967. Polyneuropathy after neurosedyn (thalidomide) and its prognosis. *Acta. Neur. Scand.* 43 Suppl. 32.

Kelsey, F. O. 1967. Events after thalidomide. *J. Dent. Res.* 46:1201.

Lasagna, L. 1960. Thalidomide — a new non-barbiturate sleep-inducing drug. *J. Chron. Dis.* 11:627.

Lenz, W. 1966. Malformations caused by drugs in pregnancy. *Am. J. Dis. Child.* 112:99.

Mellin, G. W.; and Katzenstein, M. 1962. The saga of thalidomide. *N. Eng. J. Med.* 267:1184.

Sjostrom, H. and Nilsson, R. 1972. *Thalidomide and the Power of the Drug Companies.* Penguin.

Taussig, H. B. The evils of camouflage as illustrated by thalidomide. *N. Eng. J. Med.* 269:92.

―――. 1962. A study of the German outbreak of phocomelia. *JAMA* 180:1106.

―――. 1962. Thalidomide and phocomelia. *Pediat.* 30:654.

―――. 1962. The thalidomide syndrome. *Sci. Amer.* 207, 1:20.

Visscher, M. B. 1967. New Drugs: The tortuous road to approval. Letter in *Science* 156:313.

Another Reducing Pill — High Blood Pressure in the Lungs

Brunner, H.; and Stepanek, J. 1971. Effects of aminorex on the pulmonary circulation of the dog. *Proc. Eur. Soc. Drug Toxic.* 12:123.

Doll, R. 1971. Unwanted effects of drugs. *Brit. Med. Bull.* 27:25.

Lancet. 1971. An epidemic of pulmonary hypertension. Editorial 2:252.

Greiser, E.; and Gahl, K. 1971. Frequency estimations of ingestion of aminorex and incidence of primary pulmonary hypertension in a defined population. *Proc. Eur. Soc. Study Drug Toxic.* 12:89.

Gurtner, H. P. 1971. Hypertensive pulmonary vascular disease, some remarks on its incidence and etiology. *Proc. Eur. Soc. Study Drug Toxic.* 12:81.

Lullman, H.; and Seiler, K. U. 1971. Epidemic of pulmonary hypertension. *Lancet* 2:1041.

Another Synthetic Hormone — Cancer of Vagina in Daughters

Aldrich, J. O.; Henderson, B. E.; and Townsend, D. E. 1972. Diagnostic procedures for the stilbestrol-adenosis-carcinoma syndrome. *N. Eng. J. Med.* 287:934.

Cutler, B. S.; Forbes, A. P.; Ingersoll, F. M.; and Scully, R. E. 1972. Endometrial carcinoma after stilbestrol therapy in gonadal dysgenesis. *N. Eng. J. Med.* 287:628.

British Medical Journal. 1971. Stilbestrol and cancer. Editorial 3:593.

New England Journal of Medicine. 1971. Transplacental carcinogenesis by stilbestrol. Editorial 285:404.

Greenwald, P.; Barlow, J. J.; Nasca, P. C.; and Burnett, W. S. 1971. Vaginal cancer after maternal treatment with synthetic estrogens. *N. Eng. J. Med.* 285:390.

Henderson, B. E.; Benton, B. D.; and Weaver, P. T.; *et al.* 1973. Stilbestrol and urogenital tract cancer in adolescents. *N. Eng. J. Med.* 288:354.

Herbst, A. L. 1973. Stilbestrol and vaginal cancer in young women. *Cancer* 22:292.

Herbst, A. L.; Kurman, R. J.; Scully, R. E. 1972. Vaginal and cervical abnormalities after exposure to stilbestrol *in utero*. *Obstet. and Gyn.* 40:287.

Herbst, A. L.; Kurman, R. J.; Scully, R. E.; and Poskanzer, D. C. 1972. Clear-cell adenocarcinoma of the genital tract in young females. *N. Eng. J. Med.* 287:1259.

Herbst, A. L.; and Scully, R. E. 1970. Adenocarcinoma of vagina in adolescence. *Cancer* 25:745.

Herbst, A. L.; Ulfelder, H.; and Poskanzer, D. C. 1971. Association of maternal stilbestrol therapy with tumor appearance in young women. *New Eng. J. Med.* 284:878.

Australian Drug Evaluation Committee. 1972. Stilbestrol and Adenocarcinoma of the vagina. Statement in *Med. J. Aust.* 2:622.

Wynder, E. L.; Escher, G. C.; and Mantel, N. 1966. An epidemiological investigation of cancer of the endometrium. *Cancer* 19:489.

Chapter Four   Overdose

Oxygen — An Epidemic of Blindness in Premature Infants

Ashton, N.; Ward, B.; and Serpell, G. 1953. Role of oxygen in the genesis of retrolental fibroplasia; a preliminary report. *Brit. J. Ophthal.* 37:513.

Baum, J. D.; and Tizard, J. P. M. 1970. Retrolental fibroplasia: management of oxygen therapy. *Brit. Med. Bull.* 26:171.

Campbell, K. 1951. Intensive oxygen therapy as a possible cause of retrolental fibroplasia: clinical approach. *Med. J. Austral.* 2:48.

Gyllensten, L. V.; and Hellstrom, B. E. 1956. The effects of gradual and of rapid transfer from concentrated oxygen to normal air on the oxygen-induced changes in young mice. *Amer. J. Ophthal.* 41:619.

Hepner, W. P.; Krause, A. C.; and Nardin, H. E. 1950. Retrolental fibroplasia (encephalo-ophthalmic dysplasia); study of 66 cases. *Pediat.* 5:771.

Kinsey, V. E.; Zacharias, Z. 1949. Retrolental fibroplasia: incidence in different localities in recent years and correlation of incidence with treatment given infants. *JAMA* 139:572.

Nichols, C. W.; and Lambersten, C. J. 1969. Medical progress — effects of high oxygen pressures on the eye. *N. Eng. J. Med.* 281:25.

Patz, A. 1969. Retrolental fibroplasia. *Surv. Ophthal.* 14:1.

————. 1957. The role of oxygen in retrolental fibroplasia. *Pediat.* 19:504.

Terry, T. L. 1942. Extreme prematurity and fibroblastic overgrowth of persistent vascular sheath behind each crystalline lens. *Amer. J. Ophthal.* 25:203.

————. 1945. Ocular maldevelopment in extremely premature infants; retrolental fibroplasia; general consideration. *JAMA* 128:582.

Vitamin D — High Blood Calcium

Avioli, L. V.; and Haddad, J. G. 1973. Progress in endocrinology and metabolism. Vitamin D: current concepts. *Metabolism* 22:507.

Bicknell, F.; and Prescott, F. 1953. *The Vitamins in Medicine.* London: Wm. Heinemann Medical Books Ltd.

Bills, C. E. 1935. Physiology of sterols including vitamin D. *Physiol. Rev.* 15:1.

Black, J. A.; and Bonham-Carter, R. E. 1963. Association between aortic stenosis and facies of severe infantile hypercalcemia. *Lancet* 2:745.

Bransby, E. R.; Berry, W. T. C.; and Taylor, D. M. 1964. Study of the vitamin D intakes of infants in 1960. *Brit. Med. J.* 1:1661.

Debre, R. 1948. Toxic effects of overdosage of vitamin D in children. *Amer. J. Dis. Child.* 75:787.

British Medical Journal. 1960. Aetiology of idiopathic hypercalcemia. Editorial 1:334.

F.D.A. Drug Bulletin: December 1973.

Fanconi, G.; and Girardet, P. 1952. *Familiarer persistierender phosphat-diabetes mit D-vitamin — sesistenter rachitis. Helv. Paediat. Acta.* 7:314.

Friedman, W. F.; and Roberts, W. C. 1966. Vitamin D and the supra-valvar aortic stenosis syndrome: the transplacental effects of vitamin D on the aorta of the rabbit. *Circ.* 34:77.

Goodenday, L. S.; and Gordon, G. S. 1971. No risk from vitamin D in pregnancy. *Ann. Int. Med.* 75:807.

Jeans, P. C. 1938. The effect of vitamin D on linear growth in infancy: the effect of intakes above 1,800 USP units daily. *J. Pediat.* 13:730.

————. 1950. Vitamin D. Council on food and nutrition. *JAMA* 143:177.

Joseph, M. C.; and Parrott, D. 1958. Severe infantile hypercalcemia with special reference to facies. *Arch. Dis. Child.* 33:385.

Lightwood, R. C. 1952. Idiopathic hypercalcemia with failure to thrive. *Arch. Dis. Child.* 27:302.

MacIntyre, I., ed. 1972. *Clinics in Endocrinology and Metabolism.* Philadelphia: W. B. Saunders. p. 305.

Ministry of Health. 1957. Report of the joint subcommittee on welfare foods. London: H.M.S.O.

Oppe, T. E. 1964. Infantile hypercalcemia, nutritional rickets, and infantile scurvy in Great Britain. *Brit. Med. J.* 1:1659.

Park, E. A. 1938. The use of vitamin D preparations in the prevention and treatment of disease. *JAMA* 111:1179.

Sebrell, W. H. Jr.; Harris, R. S.; and editors. 1971. *The Vitamins.* London and New York: Academic Press. p. 297.

Taussig, H. B. 1966. Possible injury to the cardiovascular system from vitamin D. *Ann. Int. Med.* 65:1195.

Verner, J. V., Jr.; Engel, F. L.; and McPherson, H. T. 1958. Vitamin D intoxication: report of two cases treated with cortisone. *Ann. Int. Med.* 48:765.

Another Headache Powder — An Epidemic of Kidney Disease

Abel, J. A. 1971. Analgesic nephropathy — a review of the literature 1967-70. *Clin. Pharm. and Therap.* 12:583.

Boyle, J. A.; and Buchanan, W. W. 1971. *Clinical Rheumatology.* Oxford: Blackwell Scientific Publications. p. 172.

Fordham, C. C. III; Huffines, W. D.; and Welt, L. G. 1965. Phenacetin-induced renal disease in rats. *Ann. Int. Med.* 62:738.

Gault, M. H.; Blennerhassett, J.; and Muehrcke, R. C. 1971. Analgesic nephropathy. *Amer. J. Med.* 51:740.

Goodman, L. S.; and Gilman, A. 1970. *The Pharmacological Basis of Therapeutics.* 4th. ed. New York: Macmillan Co. p. 329.

Kincaid-Smith, P. 1969. Analgesic nephropathy. *Med. J. Austral.* 2:1131.

Murray, R. M. 1972. Analgesic nephropathy: removal of phenacetin from proprietary analgesics. *Brit. Med. J.* 4:131.

Nanra, R. S.; and Kincaid-Smith, P. 1970. Papillary necrosis in rats caused by aspirin and aspirin-containing mixtures. *Brit. Med. J.* 3:559.

Nordonfelt, O. 1972. Deaths from renal failure in abusers of phenacetin-containing drugs. *Acta. Med. Scand.* 191:11.

Prescott, L. F. 1966. Nephrotoxicity of analgesics. *J. Pharmacol.* 18:331.

Shelley, J. H. 1967a. Phenacetin through the looking-glass. *Clin. Pharmacol. Ther.* 8:427.

—————. 1967b. Two thousand cases of renal disease due to abuse of phenacetin. *Clin. Pharmacol. Ther.* 8:427.

Spuhler, O.; and Zollinger, H. U. 1950. *Die chronische-interstitielle nephritis. Helv. Med. Acta.* 17:564.

A Diarrhea Remedy — Paralysis

Cambier, J.; Masson, M.; Berkman, N.; et al. 1972. *Neuropathie sensitive et névrite optique après absorption prolongée de chloroïdoquinone. Nouv. Presse Méd.* 1:1991.

Goodman, L. S.; and Gilman, A. 1970. *The Pharmacological Basis of Therapeutics.* 4th ed. New York: Macmillan Co. p. 1137.

Kono, R. 1971. Subacute myelo-optico-neuropathy, a new neurological disease prevailing in Japan. *Japan J. Med. Sci. Biol.* 24:195.

Nakae, K.; Yamamoto, S.; Shigematsu, I.; et al. 1973. Relation between subacute myelo-optic nueropathy (S.M.O.N.) and clioquinol: nationwide survey. *Lancet* 1:171.

Pannekoek, J. H. 1972. *Neutroxishe verschijnselen na clioquinol (enterovioform). Ned. Tijdschr. Geneeskd.* 116:1611.

Scheer, S. C. 1973. Clioquinol, Iodochlorohydroyquin. *Ann. Int. Med.* 78:309.

Year Book of Drug Therapy. 1973. p. 222.

An Inhalant for Asthma — Sudden Death

Collins, J. M.; Devitt, D. G.; Shanks, R. G.; and Swanton, J. G. 1969. The cardiotoxicity of isoprenaline during hypoxia. *Brit. J. Pharmacol.* 36:35.

Committee on Safety of Drugs. 1967. *Aerosols in Asthma.* London: (Adverse Reactions Series No. 5).

Doll, R. 1971. Unwanted effects of drugs. *Brit. Med. Bull.* 27:25.

British Medical Journal. 1972. Asthma deaths: a question answered. Editorial 4:443.

Greenberg, M. J. 1965. Isoprenaline in myocardial failure. *Lancet* 2:442.

Greenberg, M. J.; and Pines, A. 1967. Pressurized aerosols in asthma. *Brit. Med. J.* 1:563.

Heaf, P. J. D. 1970. Deaths in asthma: a therapeutic misadventure? *Brit. Med. Bull.* 26:245.

Inman, W. H. W.; and Adelstein, A. M. 1969. Rise and fall of asthma mortality in England and Wales in relation to use of pressurized aerosols. *Lance.* 2:7615.

184

Lehr, D. 1972. Isoproterenol and sudden death of asthmatic patients. *N. Eng. J. Med.* 287:987.

McManis, A. G. 1964. Incompatability between adrenalin and isoproterenol. *Med. J. Austr.* 2:76.

Smith, J. M. 1966. Death from asthma. *Lancet* 1:1042.

Speizer, F. E.; and Doll, R. 1968. A century of asthma deaths in young people. *Brit. Med. J.* 3:245.

Speizer, F. E.; Doll, R.; and Heaf, P. 1968. Observations on recent increase in mortality from asthma. *Brit. Med. J.* 1:335.

Speizer, F. E.; Doll, R.; Heaf, P.; and Strang, L. B. 1968. Investigation into use of drugs preceding death from asthma. *Brit. Med. J.* 1:339.

Stolley, P. D. 1972. Asthma mortality: why the United States was spared an epidemic of deaths due to asthma. *Amer. Rev. Resp. Dis.* 105:883.

Taylor, G. V.; and Harris, W. S. 1970. Cardiac toxicity of aerosol propellants. *JAMA* 214:81.

Chapter Five   Possible Errors — Not Proven

Removal of the Sympathetic Nerves for High Blood Pressure

Allen, E. V.; and Adson, A. W. 1940. Treatment of hypertension; medical versus surgical. *Ann. of Int. Med.* 14:288.

Evelyn, K. A.; Singh, M. M.; Chapman, W. P.; Perea, G. A.; and Thaler, H. 1960. Effect of thoracolumbar sympathectomy on the clinical course of primary (essential) hypertension. *Amer. J. Med.* 28:188.

Rowntree, L. G.; and Adson, A. W. 1925. Bilateral lumbar sympathetic neurectomy in the treatment of malignant hypertension. *JAMA* 85:959.

Smithwick, R. H.; and Thompson, J. E. 1953. Spanchnicectomy for essential hypertension; results in 1,266 cases. *JAMA* 152:1501.

Tcherdakoff, P.; Vaysse, J.; Lacombe, M.; Duden, P.; Mourad, J.; Tarrette, F.; and Melluz, P. 1966. The present status of symptomatic surgical treatment for arterial hypertension. In *Antihypertensive therapy, principles and practice; an international symposium.* ed. F. Gross with the assistance of S. R. Naegelli and A. H. Kirkwood. New York: Springer. 1966. (Symposium held June 28-July 3, 1965, sponsored by CIBA.)

White, J. C.; Smithwick, R. H.; and Simeone, F. A. 1952. *The Autonomic Nervous System.* London: Henry Kimpton.

A Pain Reliever for Arthritis

Babior, B. M.; and Davidson, C. S. 1966. Hepatitis — drug or viral? *Amer. J. Med.* 41:491.

Carver, D. H.; and Seto, D. S. 1973. Current concepts concerning the hepatitis viruses. *Pediat.* 51:115.

DiPalma, J. R., ed. 1971. *Drill's Pharmacology in Medicine.* New York: McGraw-Hill.

Journal of the American Medical Association. 1941. Present status of cinchophen and neocinchophen. Editorial 117:1182.

Hueper, W. C. 1948. Cinchophen (Atophan) A critical review. *Medicine* 27:43.

Palmer, W. L.; and Woodall, P. S. 1936. Cinchophen — is there a safe method of administration? *JAMA* 107:760.

Anticoagulants in Coronary Heart Disease

Borden, C. W. 1972. Current status of therapy with anticoagulants. *Med. Clin. N. Amer.* 56:235.

Douglas, A. S. 1969. Current status of anticoagulant treatment. In *Recent Advances in Blood Coagulation.* L. Poller, ed. London: Churchill. p. 107.

Ebert, R. V. 1972. Use of anticoagulants in acute myocardial infarction. *Circ.* 45:903.

Gifford, R. H.; and Feinstein, A. R. 1969. A critique of methodology in studies of anticoagulant therapy for acute myocardial infarction. *New Eng. J. Med.* 280:351.

Gross, H.; Vaid, A. K.; Levine, H. S.; and Asson, J. 1972. Anticoagulant therapy in myocardial infarction: an overview of methodolgy. *Amer. J. Med.* 52:421.

Hirsh, J.; Cade, J. F.; and Gallus, A. S. 1972. Anticoagulants in pregnancy: a review of indications and complications. *Amer. Heart J.* 83:301.

Hurst, J. W.; and Logue, R. B. 1970. *The Heart.* New York: McGraw-Hill. p. 991.

Wright, I. S.; Marple, C. D.; and Beck, D. F. 1948a. Report of committee for evaluation of anticoagulants in treatment of coronary thrombosis with myocardial infarction (progress report on statistical analysis of first 800 cases studied by this committee). *Amer. Heart J.* 36:801.

―――. 1948b. Anticoagulant therapy of coronary thrombosis with myocardial infarction. *JAMA* 138:1074.

Barrie, M.; Fox, W.; Weatherall, M.; and Wilkinson, M.I.P. 1968. Analysis of symptoms of patients with headaches and their response to treatment with ergot derivatives. *Quart. J. Med. NS.* 37, 146:319.

Dunlop, D. 1969. The therapeutics of migraine. In *Background to Migraine.* Smith, R., ed. London: Wm. Heinemann, Medical Books p. 72.

Friedman, A. P.; and Elkind, A. H. 1963. Appraisal of methysergide in treatment of vascular headaches of migraine types. *JAMA* 184:125.

Friedman, A. P.; Losin, S. 1961. Evaluation of UML-491 in treatment of vascular headaches. *Archiv. Neurol.* 4:241.

Graham, J. R. 1967. Inflammatory fibrosis associated with methysergide therapy. *Res. Clin. Stud. Headache.* 1:123.

———. 1964. Methysergide for prevention of headache. *New Eng. J. Med.* 270:67.

Graham, J. R.; Suby, H. I.; LeCompte, P. R.; and Sadowsky, N. L. 1966. Fibrotic disorders associated with methysergide therapy for headache. *New Eng. J. Med.* 274:359.

Hay, K. M. 1971. Migraine in general practice. In *Background to Migraine.* Cumings, J., ed. London: Wm. Heinemann Medical Books Ltd. p. 25.

Rees, W. F. 1971. Psychiatric and psychological aspects of migraine. In *Background to Migraine.* Cumings, J. N., ed. London: Wm. Heinemann Medical Books Ltd. p. 45.

Richter, A. M.; and Banker, U. P. 1973. Carotid ergotism, a complication of migraine therapy. *Radiol.* 106:339.

Sachs, O. W. 1970. *Migraine.* London: Faber and Faber, pp. 260-7.

Sicuteri, F. 1959. Prophylactic and therapeutic properties of 1-methyllysergic acid butandamide in migraine. *Int. Arch. Allergy.* 15:300.

Slugg, P. H.; and Kunkel, R. S. 1970. Complications of methysergide therapy. *JAMA* 213:297.

Waters, W. E. 1971. Epidemiological aspects of migraine. In *Background to Migraine,* Cumings, J. N. ed. London: Wm. Heinemann Medical Books Ltd. p. 37.

Acknowledgements

In the writing of this book I had much help, and owe thanks to many people.

In its preparation I was assisted by friends and colleagues on both sides of the Atlantic. (There was no simple, direct way of looking up the various errors of treatment.) The helpful suggestions of my colleagues helped me to include items that I would not have otherwise known of; their criticisms prevented me from citing those which were not mistakes. None of my colleagues are, of course, in any way responsible for what I have written.

The English colleagues who helped included Professor Colin Dollery, Professor John Goodwin, Dr. Colin Berry, Dr. John Greeve, Dr. Gerald Graham, Professor Edwin Clark, Dr. Jane Sommerville, Dr. Catherine Hallidie-Smith, Dr. Kevin O'Malley, and Dr. Lawson MacDonald.

The American colleagues were Dr. Max Landsberger, Dr. Frederick Neuburger, Dr. Erwin Neter, Dr. Alexander Nadas, Dr. Helen Taussig, Dr. Peter Vlad, Dr. Henry Wagner, Mr. S. Subramanian, Dr. Erika Bruck, Dr. Sumner Yaffe, Dr. Rita Smythe, and Dr. Sheila Mitchel.

Dr. Erwin Neter and Dr. Alexander Nadas carefully read the initial manuscript and offered detailed criticisms and suggestions, as well as much sorely needed encouragement. Professor John Goodwin was of particular help in his advice regarding historical points and in giving me wise counsel.

My debt includes others. The State University of New York at Buffalo and Dr. Jean Cortner, Chairman of the Department of Pediatrics, of which I am a member, granted me a sabbatical leave of absence, which enabled me to research and write this book, as well as to enjoy the intellectual stimulation of the University of London and the Hammersmith Postgraduate Hospital.

I owe gratitude to the staff of the Library of the Royal Society of Medicine in London, who were unfailingly courteous and helpful, and who do so much to make that great institution a delightful place to work. My thanks also go to Miss Sandra Anderson, former Chief Librarian of the Children's Hospital, who gave me special assistance.

Two able and amiable secretaries, Sandra Hafstad and Elizabeth Peery, typed and re-typed, copied and re-copied, cheerfully and without complaint. Elizabeth Peery corrected my grammar and punctuation, and made many much-needed changes.

Harry Wheeler, a charming, agreeable man with a true feeling for expression, helped to give this manuscript coherence and to make it understandable to the general reader.

Finally, and most importantly, my wife, who gave me unfailing encouragement, sacrificed many pleasant weekends and holidays, struggled with my difficult scribblings, offered innumerable helpful suggestions, and typed, and typed, and typed the initial draft.